# NO MUD, NO LOTUS

# NO MUD, NO LOTUS

## THE ART OF TRANSFORMING SUFFERING

## THICH NHAT HANH

**ALEPH**

**ALEPH**

ALEPH BOOK COMPANY
An independent publishing firm
promoted by *Rupa Publications India*

First published by Parallax Press in 2014

Published in India in 2017
by Aleph Book Company
7/16 Ansari Road, Daryaganj
New Delhi 110 002

Foreword copyright © Shantum Seth 2017
Edited by Rachel Neumann
Author photo courtesy: Ahimsa Trust
Cover image by Ton Tonic

ISBN: 978-93-84067-48-9

1 3 5 7 9 10 8 6 4 2

For sale in South Asia only

Printed and bound in India by

*Most people are afraid of suffering. But suffering
is a kind of mud to help the lotus flower of happiness grow.
There can be no lotus flower without the mud.*

—Thich Nhat Hanh

# CONTENTS

## FOREWORD

Many years ago, after burning out from political activism, in my search for a spiritual teacher who could guide me on how to 'be peace' rather than 'fight for peace', I arrived at a retreat for artists at the Ojai Foundation in California. In the five days that Thich Nhat Hanh taught there, I felt for the first time that rather than merely having a concept or notion of peace, I truly *experienced* peace. Each day we walked in meditative awareness among the sage bushes in the foothills of the Los Padres mountain, ate meals in silence, contemplated existential questions and learnt how to live happily in the present moment.

Thay (as he is known to his students—it is pronounced like the first half of 'Thailand') taught by his example, his metaphors and his practical, poetic, philosophical words. He taught us to cultivate the energy of mindfulness which would allow us, even in the most mundane of activities, to touch the miracle of life in the present moment.

When I returned home, I wrote him a letter to say that if he was interested in visiting India I would be happy to arrange something for him. As it happened, he had been planning to make a pilgrimage, 'In the Footsteps of the Buddha', and he requested me to organize this journey. It was in those thirty-five days of travel in close proximity that I came to see that I had found my spiritual guide, someone who blended everyday activities with a spiritual significance, someone who epitomized 'Engaged Buddhism'. His insights allowed me to link my inner practice to my outer social, political and ecological concerns. As I discovered, I was not the only one whom he had affected in this way.

Thay had been instrumental in influencing Martin Luther King Jr. to come out against the war in Vietnam (which is Thay's homeland); in fact, King nominated him for the Nobel Peace prize in 1967, a year when it was not conferred on anyone. His Holiness the Dalai Lama said about Thay that 'he shows us the connection between a person's inner peace and peace on earth'. He has been revolutionary, being one of the first monks in Vietnam to ride a bicycle, to change the language of liturgy from classical Chinese to Vietnamese, to bring much greater gender equity in the Buddhist sangha (community), and even to introduce practices such as hugging meditation in order to make the Dharma more accessible to Americans. Unique in many ways, Thich Nhat Hanh was once described by another Zen master, Richard Baker Roshi, as a cross between a cloud, a snail and a piece of heavy machinery.

On the actual path of the Buddha, Thay allowed me to understand the Buddha as a human being: one who had struggled with the existential questions of his time and discovered a path of awakening. Thay suggested that I continue this practice of pilgrimage that the Buddha had suggested; it would help me to understand the Buddha and his teachings better. Each winter since 1988, I have gone on pilgrimage along the path of the Buddha, and at some time during each year I have gone on retreat with Thich Nhat Hanh.

As I got to know the Buddha better, he struck me as having been a practical man, whose core teachings were ways to overcome suffering and attain happiness, peace and liberation. His concerns were rooted in our human experience, and not in metaphysical speculations on the existence of God or questions about eternity.

His discovery of the non-self and inter-dependent nature of reality—for which Thich Nhat Hanh coined the word 'inter-being'—and his teaching that this understanding can be gained by one's own effort through the practices of mindfulness, concentration and insight, were revolutionary at the time. They continue to be counter-intuitive in a world where so much emphasis is placed on individuality and the self.

Thich Nhat Hanh has taken the ancient teachings of the Buddha, developed in India 2,600 years ago, and made them relevant to our time. The perennial questions of what binds us to suffering and what can give us a sense of inner freedom and awakening remain; but the means of practice have been skilfully adapted. Thich Nhat Hanh has taken many of the practices out of the monastaries and secularized them for an everyday audience. His school of Zen Buddhism, rooted in the 'Mind Only' (Vijñānavāda) School of Mahayana Buddhism, speaks about 'Store Consciousness' which holds many seeds, both wholesome and unwholesome. The basis of Thay's practice is to water the seeds of mindfulness, thereby becoming aware of our mental formations as they arise. In this way we become aware of the roots of those mental states and, in an internal weeding of our mind's garden, we cull or transform the unwholesome seeds and cultivate or quicken the wholesome ones.

Thay has made the Buddha Dharma accessible to people from all walks of life, among them teachers, psychotherapists, lawyers, businessmen and -women, prisoners, parents and children. This has helped build a worldwide community of practitioners, both lay and monastic. In India, besides having regular gatherings of practitioners, we hold retreats and 'Days of Mindfulness', especially in the field of education and applied ethics.

Thay's simple yet articulate exposition and explanation of complex concepts makes him an artist with words. His poetry speaks eloquently to our hearts and minds. His deceptively simple teachings help make such simple acts as smiling and conscious breathing into practices of self-calming and of deep seeing.

Shantum Seth
New Delhi
August 2017

*No Mud, No Lotus*

1

THE ART OF
TRANSFORMING
SUFFERING

~

We all want to be happy and there are many books and teachers in the world that try to help people be happier. Yet we all continue to suffer.

Therefore, we may think that we're 'doing it wrong.' Somehow we are 'failing at happiness.' That isn't true. Being able to enjoy happiness doesn't require that we have zero suffering. In fact, the art of happiness is also the art of suffering well. When we learn to acknowledge, embrace, and understand our suffering, we suffer much less. Not only that, but we're also able to go further and transform our suffering into understanding, compassion, and joy for ourselves and for others.

One of the most difficult things for us to accept is that there is no realm where there's only happiness and there's no suffering. This doesn't mean that we should despair. Suffering can be transformed. As soon as we open our mouth to say 'suffering,' we know that the opposite of suffering is already there as well. Where there is suffering, there is happiness.

According to the creation story in the biblical book of Genesis, God said, 'Let there be light.' I like to imagine that light replied, saying, 'God, I have to wait for my twin brother, darkness, to be with me. I can't be there without the darkness.' God asked, 'Why do you need to wait? Darkness is there.' Light answered, 'In that case, then I am also already there.'

If we focus exclusively on pursuing happiness, we may regard suffering as something to be ignored or resisted. We think of it as something that gets in the way of happiness. But the art of happiness is also and at the same time the art of knowing how to suffer well. If we know how to use our suffering, we can transform it and suffer much less. Knowing how to suffer well is essential to realizing true happiness.

# Suffering And Happiness Are Not Separate

When we suffer, we tend to think that suffering is all there is at that moment, and happiness belongs to some other time or place. People often ask, 'Why do I have to suffer?' Thinking we should be able to have a life without any suffering is as deluded as thinking we should be able to have a left side without a right side. The same is true of thinking we have a life in which no happiness whatsoever is to be found. If the left says, 'Right, you have to go away. I don't want you. I only want the left'—that's nonsense, because then the left would have to stop existing as well. If there's no right, then there's no left. Where there is no suffering, there can be no happiness either, and vice versa.

If we can learn to see and skillfully engage with both the presence of happiness and the presence of suffering, we will go in the direction of enjoying life more. Every day we go a little farther in that direction, and eventually we realize that suffering and happiness are not two separate things.

Cold air can be painful if you aren't wearing enough warm clothes. But when you're feeling overheated or you're walking outside with proper clothing, the bracing sensation of cold air can be a source of feeling joy and aliveness. Suffering isn't some kind of external, objective source of oppression and pain. There might be things that cause you to suffer, such as loud music or bright lights, which may bring other people joy. There are things that bring you joy that annoy other people. The rainy day that ruins your plans for a picnic is a boon for the farmer whose field is parched.

Happiness is possible right now, today—but happiness cannot be without suffering. Some people think that in order to be happy they must avoid all suffering, and so they are constantly vigilant, constantly worrying. They end up sacrificing all their spontaneity, freedom, and joy. This isn't correct. If you can recognize and accept your pain without running away from it, you will discover that although pain is there, joy can also be there at the same time.

Some say that suffering is only an illusion or that to live wisely we have to 'transcend' both suffering and joy. I say the opposite. The way to suffer well and be happy is to stay in touch with what is actually going on; in doing so, you will gain liberating insights into the true nature of suffering *and* of joy.

## No Mud, No Lotus

Both suffering and happiness are of an organic nature, which means they are both transitory; they are always changing. The flower, when it wilts, becomes the compost. The compost can help grow a flower again. Happiness is also organic and impermanent by nature. It can become suffering and suffering can become happiness again.

If you look deeply into a flower, you see that a flower is made only of nonflower elements. In that flower there is a cloud. Of course we know a cloud isn't a flower, but without a cloud, a flower can't be. If there's no cloud, there's no rain, and no flower can grow. You don't have to be a dreamer to see a cloud floating in a flower. It's really there. Sunlight is also there. Sunlight isn't flower, but without sunlight no flower is possible.

If we continue to look deeply into the flower, we see many other things, like the earth and the minerals. Without them a flower cannot be. So it's a fact that a flower is made only of nonflower elements. A flower can't be by herself alone. A flower can only inter-be with everything else. You can't remove the sunlight, the soil, or the cloud from the flower.

In each of our Plum Village practice centers around the world, we have a lotus pond. Everyone knows we need to have mud for lotuses to grow. The mud doesn't smell so good, but the lotus flower smells very good. If you don't have mud, the lotus won't manifest. You can't grow lotus flowers on marble. Without mud, there can be no lotus.

It is possible of course to get stuck in the 'mud' of life. It's easy enough to notice mud all over you at times. The hardest thing to practice is not allowing yourself to be overwhelmed by despair. When you're overwhelmed by despair, all you can see is suffering everywhere you look. You feel as if the worst thing is happening to you. But we must remember that suffering is a kind of mud that we need in order to generate joy and happiness. Without suffering, there's no happiness. So we shouldn't discriminate against the mud. We have to learn how to embrace and cradle our own suffering and the suffering of the world, with a lot of tenderness.

When I lived in Vietnam during the war, it was difficult to see our way through that dark and heavy mud. It seemed like the destruction would just go on and on forever. Every day people would ask me if I thought the war would end soon. It was very difficult to answer, because there was no end in sight. But I knew if I said, 'I don't know,' that would only water their seeds of despair. So when people asked me that question, I replied, 'Everything is impermanent, even war. It will end some day.' Knowing that, we could continue to work for peace. And indeed the war did end. Now the former mortal enemies are busily trading and touring back and forth, and people throughout the world enjoy practicing our tradition's teachings on mindfulness and peace.

If you know how to make good use of the mud, you can grow beautiful lotuses. If you know how to make good use of suffering, you can produce happiness. We do need some suffering to make happiness possible. And most of us have enough suffering inside and around us to be able to do that. We don't have to create more.

## Did The Buddha Suffer

When I was a young monk, I believed that the Buddha didn't suffer once he had become enlightened. Naively I asked myself, 'What's the use of becoming a Buddha if you continue to suffer?' The Buddha did suffer, because he had a body, feelings, and perceptions, like all of us. Sometimes he probably had a headache. Sometimes he suffered from rheumatism. If he happened to eat something not well cooked, then he had intestinal problems. So he suffered physically, and he suffered emotionally as well. When one of his beloved students died, he suffered. How can you not suffer when a dear friend has just died? The Buddha wasn't a stone. He was a human being. But because he had a lot of insight, wisdom, and compassion, he knew how to suffer and so he suffered much less.

## The Four Noble Truths

The very first teaching the Buddha gave after his enlightenment was about suffering. It's called the Four Noble Truths. The

Buddha's Four Noble Truths are: there is suffering; there is a course of action that generates suffering; suffering ceases (i.e., there is happiness); and there is a course of action leading to the cessation of suffering (the arising of happiness).

When you first hear that suffering is a Noble Truth, you might wonder what's so noble about suffering? The Buddha was saying that if we can recognize suffering, and if we embrace it and look deeply into its roots, then we'll be able to let go of the habits that feed it and, at the same time, find a way to happiness. Suffering has its beneficial aspects. It can be an excellent teacher.

## What Suffering Is Made Of

There is the suffering of the body, including the sensations of pain, illness, hunger, and physical injury. Some of this suffering is simply unavoidable. Then there is the suffering of the mind, including anxiety, jealousy, despair, fear, and anger. We have the seeds, the potential in us for understanding, love, compassion, and insight, as well as the seeds of anger, hate, and greed. While we can't avoid all the suffering in life, we can suffer much less by not watering the seeds of suffering inside us.

Are you at war with your body? Do you neglect or punish your body? Have you truly gotten to know your body? Can you feel at home with your body? Suffering can be either physical or mental or both, but every kind of suffering manifests somewhere in the body and creates tension and stress. We are told that we should release the tension in our body. Many of us have tried very hard! We want to release the tension in our body, but we can't release it. Our attempts at reducing tension in us won't work unless we first acknowledge that it's there.

When you cut your finger, you just wash it and your body knows how to heal. When a nonhuman animal living in the forest is injured, she knows what to do. She stops searching for something to eat or looking for a mate. She knows, through generations of ancestral knowledge, that it's not good for her to do so. She finds a quiet place and just lies down, doing nothing. Nonhuman animals instinctively know that stopping is the best way to get healed. They don't need a doctor, a drugstore, or a pharmacist.

We human beings used to have this kind of wisdom. But we have lost touch with it. We don't know how to rest anymore. We don't allow the body to rest, to release the tension, and heal. We rely almost entirely on medication to deal with sickness and pain. Yet the most effective ways to ease and transform our suffering are already available to us without any prescription and at no financial cost. I'm not suggesting that you should throw away all your medications. Some of us do need to use certain medicines. But we can sometimes use them in smaller quantities and to much greater effect when we know how to let our body and mind truly rest.

## Healing Medicine

The main affliction of our modern civilization is that we don't know how to handle the suffering inside us and we try to cover it up with all kinds of consumption. Retailers peddle a plethora of classic and novel devices to help us cover up the suffering inside. But unless and until we're able to face our suffering, we can't be present and available to life, and happiness will continue to elude us.

There are many people who have enormous suffering, and don't know how to handle it. For many people, it starts already at a very young age. So why don't schools teach our young people the way to manage suffering? If a student is very unhappy, he can't concentrate and he can't learn. The suffering of each of us affects others. The more we learn about the art of suffering well, the less suffering there will be in the world.

Mindfulness is the best way to be with our suffering without being overwhelmed by it. Mindfulness is the capacity to dwell in the present moment, to know what's happening in the here and now. For example, when we're lifting our two arms, we're conscious of the fact that we're lifting our arms. Our mind is with our lifting of our arms, and we don't think about the past or the future, because lifting our arms is what's happening in the present moment.

To be mindful means to be aware. It's the energy that knows what is happening in the present moment. Lifting our arms and knowing that we're lifting our arms—that's mindfulness, mindfulness of our action. When we breathe in and we know we're breathing in, that's mindfulness. When we make a step and we know that the steps are taking place, we are mindful of the steps. Mindfulness is always mindfulness of *something*. It's the energy that helps us be aware of what is happening right now and right here, in our body, in our feelings, in our perceptions, and around us.

With mindfulness, you can recognize the presence of the suffering in you and in the world. And it's with that same energy that you tenderly embrace the suffering. By being aware of your in-breath and out-breath you generate the energy of mindfulness, so you can continue to cradle the suffering.

Practitioners of mindfulness can help and support each other in recognizing, embracing, and transforming suffering. With mindfulness we are no longer afraid of pain. We can even go further and make good use of suffering to generate the energy of understanding and compassion that heals us and we can help others to heal and be happy as well.

## Generating Mindfulness

The way we start producing the medicine of mindfulness is by stopping and taking a conscious breath, giving our complete attention to our in-breath and our out-breath. When we stop and take a breath in this way, we unite body and mind and come back home to ourselves. We feel our bodies more fully. We are truly alive only when the mind is with the body. The great news is that oneness of body and mind can be realized just by one in-breath. Maybe we have not been kind enough to our body for some time. Recognizing the tension, the pain, the stress in our body, we can bathe it in our mindful awareness, and that is the beginning of healing.

If we take care of the suffering inside us, we have more clarity, energy, and strength to help address the suffering, violence, poverty, and inequity of our loved ones as well as the suffering in our community and the world. If, however, we are preoccupied with the fear and despair in us, we can't help remove the suffering of others. There is an art to suffering well. If we know how to take care of our suffering, we not only suffer much, much less, we also create more happiness around us and in the world.

*No Mud, No Lotus*

2

SAYING
HELLO

~

The first step in the art of transforming suffering is to come home to our suffering and recognize it. For most of us, there's always a mental discourse going on day and night in our heads. We relive the past, we worry about the future. We don't stop to take a breath, to even notice if we're suffering—until suddenly, seemingly out of nowhere, the suffering overwhelms us. Our thinking, perceiving, and worrying take away all the space inside us, and keep us from being in touch with what's happening moment to moment.

The Buddha said that nothing can survive without food. This is true, not just for the physical existence of living beings, but also for states of mind. Love needs to be nurtured and fed to survive; and our suffering also survives because we enable and feed it. We ruminate on suffering, regret, and sorrow. We chew on them, swallow them, bring them back up, and eat them again and again. If we're feeding our suffering while we're walking, working, eating, or talking, we are making ourselves victims of the ghosts of the past, of the future, or our worries in the present. We're not living our lives.

If we try to use consumption to ignore or distract ourselves from our suffering, we end up making the suffering worse. We turn on the television. We talk or text or gossip on the phone. We get on the Internet. We find ourselves in front of the refrigerator over and over again.

When we cut ourselves off from the pain in our mind, we're also abandoning our bodies where suffering is being stored. When we feel loneliness and despair, we seek to cover them up and pretend they're not there. We don't feel very well inside, so in order to forget, we go and look for something to eat even if we're not hungry at all. We eat in an attempt to feel better, but we end up becoming addicted to eating, because we are trying to cover up the suffering inside, and the real problem is left unaddressed. Or we may become addicted to computer games, or other kinds of audiovisual entertainment.

Electronic distractions not only fail to help heal the underlying suffering, they may contain stories or images that feed our craving, jealousy, anger, or despair. Instead of making us feel better, they numb us only briefly, then make us feel worse. To consume in order to cover up our suffering doesn't work. We need a spiritual practice to have the strength and skill to look deeply into our suffering, to get insight into it and make a breakthrough.

## Stopping And Acknowledging Suffering

When suffering arises, the first thing to do is to stop, follow our breathing, and acknowledge it. Don't try to deny uncomfortable emotions or push them down.

> *Breathing in, I know suffering is there.*
> *Breathing out, I say hello to my suffering.*

To take one mindful breath requires the presence of our mind, our body, and our intention. With our conscious breath, we reunite our body and mind and arrive in the present moment. Just breathing in mindfully already brings us a surprising amount of freedom. With each breath, we generate mindful energy, bringing mind and body together in the present moment to receive this caring acknowledgment of our suffering. In just two or three breaths taken with your full attention, you may notice that regret and sorrow about the past have paused, as well as uncertainty, fear, and worries about the future.

## Body And Mind Together

Each of us has a body, but we aren't always in touch with it. Maybe our body needs us, our body is calling us, but we don't hear it. We're so caught up in our job, our computer, our phone, or in our conversation, we can forget we even have a body.

If we can get in touch with our body, then we can also get in touch with our feelings. There are many feelings calling to us. Every feeling is like our child. Suffering is a hurt child crying out to us. But we ignore the voice of the child within.

The process of healing begins when we mindfully breathe in. In daily life, very often our body is here but our mind is off in the past, in the future, or in our projects. The mind is not with the body. When we breathe in and focus our attention on our in-breath, we reunite body and mind. We become aware of what is going on in the present moment, in our body, in our perceptions, and around us.

When we bring our mind home to our body, something wonderful happens; our mental discourse stops its chattering. Thinking can be productive, but the reality is that most of our thinking is unproductive. When we think, it may be easy for us to be lost in our thinking. But when we use our breath to bring our mind home to the body, we can stop the thinking.

When you come back to yourself and breathe mindfully, your mind's attention has only one object, your breath. If you continue to breathe in and out mindfully, you maintain that state of presence and freedom. Your mind will be clearer and you will make better decisions. It's much better to make a decision when

*No Mud, No Lotus*

your mind is clear and free rather than in the sway of fear, anger, and worries.

When I was a young monk, I believed that it took a long time to get any kind of insight. The truth is, there are insights that can come right away. When you practice mindfulness of breathing, you know right away that you are *alive,* and that to be alive is a wonder. If you can be aware that you have a living body, and notice when there's tension in your body, that's already an important insight. With that insight, you have already begun to diagnose the situation. You don't need to practice eight years or twenty years in order to wake up.

Breathing mindfully isn't something hard to do. You don't have to suffer while breathing. You're already doing it all day long. You don't need to struggle to control your breathing. In fact, breathing in can become a real pleasure. You just allow yourself to breathe in naturally while focusing your attention on your in-breath. It's like the morning sunshine on a flower that has closed overnight. The sunshine doesn't interfere with the flower. The sunshine just embraces and subtly permeates the flower. Embraced by the energy of the sunshine, the flower begins to bloom.

## The Pull Of Distractions

When we stop the busyness of the mind and come back to ourselves, the enormity and rawness of our suffering can seem very intense because we are so used to ignoring it and distracting ourselves. When we feel suffering, we have the urge to run away from it and fill ourselves up with junk food, junk entertainment, anything to keep our mind off the pain that is there inside us.

It doesn't work. We may succeed in numbing ourselves from it for a little while, but the suffering inside wants our attention and it will fester and churn away until it gets it. We run away from ourselves because we don't want to be with ourselves. Our pain is a kind of energy that is not pleasant. We fear that if we release our diversions and come back to ourselves, we'll be overwhelmed by the suffering, despair, anger, and loneliness inside. So we continue to run away. But if we don't have the time and the willingness to take care of ourselves, how can we offer any genuine care to the people we love?

That's why the first practice is to stop running, come home to our bodies, and recognize our suffering. When we notice anger or anxiety coming up, we can recognize these feelings of suffering. Suffering is one energy. Mindfulness is another energy that we can call on to come and embrace the suffering. The practice of mindful breathing is essential, because it provides us with the energy we need for the other steps of taking care of suffering.

With mindful breathing, you can recognize the presence of a painful feeling, just like an older sibling greets a younger sibling. You can say, 'Hello, my suffering. I know you are there.' In this way, the energy of mindfulness keeps us from being overwhelmed by painful feelings. We can even smile to our suffering and say, 'Good morning, my pain, my sorrow, my fear. I see you. I am here. Don't worry.'

## Embracing Suffering

If we let the suffering come up and just take over our mind, we can be quickly overwhelmed by it. So we have to invite another energy to come up at the same time, the energy of mindfulness. The function of mindfulness is, first, to recognize the suffering and then to take care of the suffering. The work of mindfulness is first to recognize the suffering and second to embrace it. A mother taking care of a crying baby naturally will take the child into her arms without suppressing, judging it, or ignoring the crying. Mindfulness is like that mother, recognizing and embracing suffering without judgment.

So the practice is not to fight or suppress the feeling, but rather to cradle it with a lot of tenderness. When a mother embraces her child, that energy of tenderness begins to penetrate into the body of the child. Even if the mother doesn't understand at first why the child is suffering and she needs some time to find out what the difficulty is, just her act of taking the child into her arms with tenderness can already bring relief. If we can recognize and cradle the suffering while we breathe mindfully, there is relief already.

Embracing our suffering may seem to be the opposite of what we want to do, especially if our suffering is very large, as with depression. Depression is one of the most widespread forms of suffering in our time. It can take away our peace, our joy, our stability, and even our ability to eat, move about, or do simple tasks. It can seem insurmountable and we may think that the only thing we can do is either to run away from it or give in to it.

But nonjudgmentally recognizing and embracing this great suffering is not at all the same thing as giving in to it. Once you have offered your acknowledgment and care to this suffering, it naturally will become less impenetrable and more workable; and then you have the chance to look into it deeply, with kindness (but still always with a solid ground of mindful breathing to support you), and find out why it has come to you. It is trying to get your attention, to tell you something, and now you can take the opportunity to listen. You can ask someone to look with you—a teacher, a friend, a psychotherapist. Whether alone or together with your friends, you can explore what kind of roots it has, and what nutriments and habits of consumption have been feeding your sorrow. You can discover how, through looking deeply, you can transform this organic 'garbage' into compost, which in turn may become many beautiful flowers of understanding, compassion, and joy.

## The Bell

Even with the best intention—and even with a longstanding mindfulness practice, we all have the tendency to run into the future or go back into the past, to search for happiness elsewhere. A bell of mindfulness, whether it is an actual bell or some other sound, is a wonderful reminder to come back to ourselves, to come back to *life* here in the present moment.

The sound of the bell is the voice of the Buddha within. Every one of us has Buddha nature—the capacity for compassionate, clear, understanding nature—within us. So when we hear the sound of the bell, if we like practicing mindfulness, we can respond to that intervention with respect and appreciation. In my tradition, every time we hear the bell, we pause. We stop moving, talking, and thinking, and we listen to the voice of the heart.

We don't say that we 'hit the bell' or 'strike the bell.' Rather, we say we 'invite the bell' to sound, because the bell is a friend, an enlightened friend that helps us wake up and guides us home to ourselves. Gentleness and nonviolence are characteristics of the sound of the bell. Its sound is gentle but very powerful.

When you hear the sound of the bell, take the opportunity to come home to yourself and enjoy your breathing. Take a few moments to inhale and exhale deeply and touch a little happiness. If you want to experience what the end of suffering will feel like, it is in the here and the now with *this* breath. If you want nirvana, it's right here.

*Breathing in, I know I am breathing in.*
*Breathing out, I smile.*

3

LOOKING
DEEPLY

~

Having embraced a child for some minutes, a caring, attentive parent often discovers the cause for his baby's suffering. Maybe the baby was hungry or had a little fever. The same is true with our suffering. After we've cradled and embraced our suffering for some time, we can look deeply into it and begin to understand what has caused it and what has been feeding it. Understanding the nature of the situation makes it much easier to transform it.

## Understanding The Pain

When we are in crisis or pain, we need to first take care of the immediate need, which is that crisis. Once our mindful energy has soothed our suffering, we can begin to look more deeply into its nature and sources. Just as when we have a headache, acknowledging its existence and understanding its causes helps us find the appropriate remedy for it, so understanding eases our pain and helps us transform it into compassion.

The important mindfulness practice of cultivating understanding means first of all understanding suffering: the suffering inside us and the suffering of others. A human being without understanding is a human being without compassion, utterly alone, cut off, and isolated. To connect with others, however, we first have to be willing to look deeply into ourselves.

## The Pain Of Our Ancestors

Some of our ill-being comes from hurt and pain in our own life; but some has been transmitted to us by our ancestors. Think of a stalk of corn that grows from a seed. Each ear of corn, each leaf, contains that initial seed. In every cell of the plant that seed is there. And just as the plant of corn is the continuation of the seed of corn, you are the continuation of your parents.

When you see a picture of yourself as a five-year-old child, you may ask yourself, 'Am I the same person as that child?' The answer isn't 'Yes' or 'No.' Your form, your feelings, your mental formations, your perceptions, and your consciousness are quite different from when you were that child. It's clear you aren't exactly that same person. But if you say that you are a completely different person, that's equally wrong. You and that young child inter-are with each other.

Before my mother gave birth to me, she had a miscarriage. The child who didn't arrive that time—was he my brother or was he me? We aren't the same, but we aren't totally different. My feet have been transmitted to me by my ancestors. When I walk, I walk with my own feet, but these feet are also theirs. I can see the hand of my mother in my hand. I can see the arms of my father in my arms. I am my parents continuation.

There are those who have lost their biological parents, or never knew them, and have no chance to connect with them in person. There are also people who grew up with their blood relatives, whose parents are still alive, yet they are unable to communicate with them. In all these situations, even if you don't have a regular interpersonal relationship with your parents or your ancestors, your body and mind contain their suffering and their hopes as well as your own.

So if you have suffering in you and you don't know where it comes from, looking deeply you may see that this is the suffering of your ancestors, handed down from one generation to another, because no one knew how to recognize, embrace, and heal it. It's not your fault, nor is it their fault.

Many people are angry at their parents because of the suffering they experienced as children. They say, 'That man, I don't want anything to do with him.' You may believe that your father is outside of you, but your father is also inside of you. Your father is present in every cell of your body. You can't remove your father from you. It's impossible. When he suffered, you suffered, and when you suffer, he suffers. Getting angry with your father, you're getting angry with yourself. The suffering of the parent is the suffering of the child. Looking deeply is a chance to transform and heal this suffering and stop the cycle.

So part of looking deeply into our suffering is to know that it is not ours alone. When we're able to embrace our suffering, we're also embracing our ancestors, and the healing goes back through the generations. When we practice mindful breathing to know how to recognize, embrace, and transform our pain, we do it for them as well as for us. Then we can heal not only our own suffering and that of our ancestors, but we can also avoid transmitting this suffering to our loved ones, to our children, and their children.

## Exploring Our Fear

One unnecessary suffering that we can let go of is the suffering of fear. So many of us walk around with the pain and agitation of useless fear, whether that is the fear of dying, fear of hunger, injury or loss, fear of what might happen if we do the wrong thing, or fear of being hurt by or of hurting someone we care about.

Many people suffer due to the fear of dying. We want to

live forever. We fear annihilation. We don't want to pass from being into non-being. This is understandable. If you believe that one day you will cease to exist altogether, it can be very scary. But if you take the time to still the activities of body and mind and look deeply, you may see that you are dying right this very moment. You think that you will die in a few years, or twenty years, or thirty years. That's not true. You are dying now. You have been dying all the time. It's actually very pleasant to die, which is also to live.

There are many cells inside your body that are dying as you read these words. Fifty to seventy billion cells die each day in the average human adult. You are too busy to organize funerals for all of them! At the very same time, new cells are being born, and you don't have the time to sing Happy Birthday to them. If old cells don't die, there's no chance for new cells to be born. So death is a very good thing. It's very crucial for birth. You are undergoing birth and death in this very moment.

While most people are intensely afraid of dying, there are also people who are weary of living. They get bored after fifty, seventy, or maybe only twenty or thirty years. They find life unbearable and are seeking nonbeing. Some of them think that suicide is a way to end the suffering and to pass from the realm of being into nonbeing. Both of these preconceptions cause suffering because they ignore the reality that life and death always go together. You can't take one out of the other. Even after your so-called death, you will continue in some way.

Deep looking can dismantle these kinds of notions. There is no birth and death; everything dies and renews itself all the time. When you get that kind of insight, you no longer tire yourself out with anxiety and aversion.

## Your True Aspiration

When we are full of fear, we are often completely focused on preventing the event we dread, and we forget that joy is also possible even in an unpredictable world. We believe that we need to obtain a certain diploma or career in order to be safe and be a success. There are people who are victims of this kind of success. They get the things they worked so hard to achieve, and then they find themselves trapped in ways they hadn't anticipated. But no one is ever a victim of his or her happiness.

Many of us live in communities where everyone has a roof over their head and enough food to eat, and no one is scared of bombs dropping on them, yet people are still suffering. This is because we have forgotten or misplaced our deepest aspiration.

Many of us slog through life without conscious awareness or intention. We set ourselves a course and we barrel ahead, without stopping to ask whether this path is fulfilling our most important goals. That's partly because many of us believe that happiness is not possible in the here and now. We think we need to struggle now so that we will be happy in the future. So we postpone happiness and try to run into the future and attain the conditions of happiness that we don't have now.

If you breathe in and bring your mind home to your body, you can recognize immediately the many conditions of happiness that you already have. You can look deeply at your true aspiration and get the insight, 'I don't need to run into the future in order to be happy.' We all have the habit of running, every one of us. That habit creates tension, not only in the body but in the mind, and it's a major source of our suffering.

Many of us believe that we can only be happy if we have

a great deal of power, fame, wealth, and sensual pleasures. But when we look around we see there are people who have plenty of these things, yet they aren't happy. These objects of desire are not real conditions of happiness. Looking deeply, we can recognize that habit energy of running and envision what things would be like if we didn't let it push us to run anymore.

Everyone has volition, a strong motivation that fuels us and, when it's a healthy one, brings us joy. When I was twelve, I knew I wanted to be a monk. At the age of sixteen, I left my mother and my family to become ordained as a novice monk. I loved my mother so much; I wanted to be near her. On the other hand, I knew my greatest happiness would be to live as a monk. I had to sacrifice the good times I would have spent with my mother and I was sad about it; but I didn't let any fear of loss hold me back, because I knew I was on the path of fulfilling my true aspiration.

If we haven't taken the time to stop, come home to ourselves, and look deeply, we may not know what brings us our deepest happiness. Perhaps we are working hard at success in one area, but our deepest aspiration is to work in another field or to help people in another way. We need to stop and ask, 'Can I realize my deepest aspiration if I pursue this path?' 'What is really preventing me from taking the path I most deeply desire?'

## Developing Understanding And Compassion

Just as the well-tended compost becomes a flower garden, when we take care of and look deeply into our sorrow, it transforms into understanding and compassion.

The way to understanding is first to listen to yourself,

because the roots of our suffering are deep and connected with the roots of the suffering of others. Usually we think that other people, such as our parents, our partner, or people at work, are to blame for our hurt. But looking more deeply, we can see the true sources of our own suffering, and we also can see that the person who we think is out to get us is a victim of his or her own suffering. Understanding our own hurt allows us to see and understand the suffering of others. Looking without judgment, we can understand, and compassion is born. Transformation is possible.

When you're upset with someone, it may seem at first that this other person has no reason to suffer. His life may seem happy and carefree, and he may have all the things in his life that you think you want. But when you are able to look deeply enough, you will see the suffering in him.

Sitting and walking mindfully, you direct your attention to the causes underlying the other person's behavior. You see clearly that he has a lot of pain inside and doesn't know how to handle it. That is why he suffers so much and makes the people around him suffer. What he needs is help, not punishment. If you stay with this practice, the sufffering of anger or jealousy in you will dissipate and the flower of compassion will be born.

When there is no more blame or criticism in your eyes, when you are able to look at others with compassion, you see things very differently. You speak differently. The other person can sense you are truly seeing her and understanding her, and that already eases her pain significantly.

Even a child can look deeply and see that his parents have difficulties and don't know how to handle their own pain. Their suffering overflows out onto the people around them, including—even especially—the ones they love. An understanding of suffering helps anger to be transformed. And when compassion is born in your heart, you naturally want to reach out, to help others suffer less.

Understanding and compassion are not for somebody else to cultivate. They can heal you and increase your happiness. A human being without understanding and compassion isn't a happy being. Without compassion and understanding, you are utterly alone and cut off. You can't relate to any other human being.

I wouldn't want to be in a world without any suffering, because then there would be no compassion and understanding either. If you haven't suffered hunger, you can't appreciate having something to eat. If you haven't gone through a war, you don't know the value of peace. That is why we should not try to run away from one unpleasant thing after another. Holding our suffering, looking deeply into it, and transforming it into compassion, we find a way to happiness.

With mindfulness, the feelings that have been painful and difficult transform into something beautiful: the wondrous, healing balm of understanding and compassion.

## Easing Communication

Our most basic difficulty is that sometimes we lack good communication inside ourselves. We don't understand ourselves. In our body there are conflicts and tensions, and we can't resolve them. Instead of stopping and looking deeply, we are running as far away as possible from the loneliness, grief, sadness, anger, and emptiness that we feel we can't bear.

If we're in this situation and we find ourselves unable to communicate well with others, that's normal. They aren't communicating with themselves, and we aren't communicating with ourselves, so is it any wonder we have difficulty communicating with each other? The situation doesn't call for blame or punishment; it calls for understanding and compassion.

With the practice of mindfulness, starting with our mindful breathing, we recognize that suffering is there in us and suffering is also there in the other person. We ourselves need help. The other person also needs help. Nobody needs punishment. So when you get angry and you suffer, don't try to say or do something to punish the other person, because there is a lot of suffering in her already, and punishing her won't improve the situation at all.

The most effective way to show compassion to another is to listen, rather than talk. You have an opportunity to practice deep, compassionate listening. If you can listen to the other person with compassion, your listening is like a salve for her wound. In the practice of compassionate listening, you listen with only one purpose, which is to give the other person the chance to speak out and to suffer less.

This practice requires steady concentration and mindful breathing in and out, to refrain from interrupting or attempting to correct what you hear. While the other person speaks, you may hear a lot of bitterness, wrong perception, and accusation in her speech. If you allow these things to touch off the anger in you, you'll lose your capacity to listen deeply.

Instead, hold on to your true purpose and remind yourself, 'Listening like this, my sole aim is to help the other person to suffer less. She may be full of wrong perceptions, but I won't interrupt her. If I jump in with my perspective on things or correct her, it will become a debate, not a practice of deep listening. Another time, there may be a chance for me to offer her a little information so that she can correct her wrong perception. But not now.' That kind of mindfulness helps you to keep your compassion alive and protects you from having the seed of anger in you touched off. Who knows, you may be the first one who has listened deeply to her like that.

When you have understood her suffering and you are ready to speak, your voice will contain compassion. You can use loving speech, free of judgment or blame. You might say something such as, 'It's not my intention to make you suffer. I didn't understand your suffering. I'm sorry. Please help me by telling me about your struggles and your difficulties. I need help in understanding you.' Or you may be able to say,' I know you have suffered a lot during the past many years. I was not able to help you to suffer less. Instead, I have made the situation worse. I have reacted with anger and stubbornness, and instead of helping you, I have made you suffer more. I am very sorry.' Many of us are no longer able to use that kind of language with the other person because we have suffered so much. But when we consciously practice deep listening and loving speech, so much healing and happiness is possible.

## Being A Mindfulness Bell For A Loved One

If you have a loved one who suffers, you can be a compassionate ally for him. You can offer to sit with him when he has to have a difficult conversation with somebody, either in person or over the phone. Every time the person he's speaking with says something that you think might trigger your loved one's anger or sadness, you can squeeze your loved one's hand. That is your bell of mindfulness. Say to your loved one ahead of time, 'When you feel that squeeze, remember you don't have to say anything. Take it as a reminder to breathe in and out three times slowly, paying attention to your breath. Try to smile. Maybe the person you are talking with will be very surprised by your quality of listening. Just breathe in and out three times, don't say anything, and try to smile.'

Play the role of a bell of mindfulness. Your squeezing the hand is like a bell, lovingly calling your friend to come back to himself. That squeeze means, 'I am here for you. You don't need to do anything but breathe.'

4

EASE

~

Some of the situations and accidents that cause us the greatest suffering, when seen objectively, do not look very big. But because we don't know how to manage them, they feel enormous. If we lose a loved one, that is of course a major loss. There is real pain there, and we feel it mightily. But we also can spend days worrying that someone doesn't like us, or that we didn't say or do the right thing, or that we won't get the promotion we want. These are small sufferings, relatively speaking, but we magnify them until they seem to take up all our mindspace.

If we know how to handle the little sufferings, we don't have to suffer on a daily basis. We can practice letting go of what the French call *les petites miseres,* the little miseries, and save our energy to embrace and soothe the true pains of illness and loss that are unavoidable.

## Releasing The Arrow

There is a Buddhist teaching found in the Sallatha Sutta, known as The Arrow. It says if an arrow hits you, you will feel pain in that part of your body where the arrow hit; and then if a second arrow comes and strikes exactly at the same spot, the pain will not be only double, it will become at least ten times more intense.

The unwelcome things that sometimes happen in life—being rejected, losing a valuable object, failing a test, getting injured in an accident—are analogous to the first arrow. They cause some pain. The second arrow, fired by our own selves, is our reaction, our storyline, and our anxiety. All these things magnify the suffering. Many times, the ultimate disaster we're ruminating upon hasn't even happened. We may worry, for example, that we have cancer and that we're going to die soon. We don't know, and our fear of the unknown makes the pain grow even bigger.

The second arrow may take the form of judgment ('how could I have been so stupid?'), fear ('what if the pain doesn't go away?'), or anger ('I hate that I'm in pain. I don't deserve this!'). We can quickly conjure up a hell realm of negativity in our minds that multiplies the stress of the actual event, by ten times or even more. Part of the art of suffering well is learning not to magnify our pain by getting carried away in fear, anger, and despair. We build and maintain our energy reserves to handle the big sufferings; the little sufferings we can let go.

If you lose your job, of course it's a normal response to feel fear and anxiety. It is true that in most cases to be out of work is a suffering; and there is real danger attached if you don't have enough to eat or can't afford necessary medicine. But you don't need to make this suffering worse by spinning stories in your head that are much worse than the reality. Some people in this situation may think 'I'm no good at this or that,' or 'I'll never get another job,' or 'I failed my family.' It's important to remember that everything is impermanent. A suffering can arise—or can work itself out—for anyone at any moment.

Instead of throwing good energy away on condemning yourself or obsessing over what catastrophes might be lurking around the corner, you can simply be present with the real suffering that is right in front of you, with what is happening right now. Mindfulness is recognizing what is there in the present moment. Suffering is there, yes; but what is also there is that you are still alive: 'Breathing in, I know I'm alive.' Your eyes still work: 'Breathing in, I'm aware of my eyes. Breathing out, I smile to my eyes.'

To have eyes in good condition is a wonderful thing. Because you have eyes in good condition, there's a paradise of shapes and colors available to you at every moment. There are those among us who have gone blind. They've lost that endlessly changing kaleidoscope of shapes and colors; and what they want more than anything is to have that faculty back again. You only need to open your eyes to be in touch with that kaleidoscope. It's a paradise, if you only stop to notice and appreciate it. If you have eyes in good condition, just open them and enjoy what you see. Happiness is possible immediately—even if not everything is perfect.

When you look at the person you love, if he or she is absorbed in anxiety, you can help that person to get out. 'Darling, do you see the sunset? Do you see the spring coming?' This is mindfulness. Mindfulness is for making us aware of what is happening now. Not only are there always conditions of happiness present in me, but they are also all around me.

## Complexes And The Sense Of A Separate Self

Most of the second arrows with which we shoot ourselves come from our beliefs. One basic problem that causes us to suffer is the idea that we are a separate self. This gives rise to the complexes of inferiority, superiority, and equality. As long as we have the idea of a self, we try to protect this self by running away from all kinds of threats and discomforts. If there is some loneliness, some anger, or some fear, we don't like it and we try to pretend that the suffering is not there. 'It's nothing,' we say, nervously trying to sweep all the feelings under the rug.

We create unnecessary pain when our reaction to an unpleasant event is to compare our self with other selves, reinforcing our illusion of separateness. We may feel a fleeting satisfaction when we tell ourselves, 'I am better than he is. I don't care what he says.' That's the complex of superiority. Or we may try to immunize ourselves from disappointment by thinking, 'I'll never be as good as she is. There's no point in trying.' That's the complex of inferiority. Most people think the best way to deal with these complexes is to maintain the belief, 'I am their equal.' But that is also a complex invented by the comparing mind.

Equality, when it refers to opportunity and access to resources, in other words treating everyone's needs and feelings with respect, is a good thing. But the constant effort to prove one's self equal to all others brings only short-lived relief from the pain of discrimination—and, ultimately, creates more suffering because it perpetuates our incorrect belief in a separate self. If we think, 'I claim the right to be as good as he is,' there is still the idea of a separate self, and therefore there will always be comparison. As long as you continue to compare, you suffer from the fear of coming up short; and, even worse, you keep yourself trapped in a constant, painful delusion of isolation and alienation.

## Greener Grass! The Story Of The Buddha And Mara

This story, about the Buddha meeting Mara, illustrates the problem with complexes. In Buddhist stories, Mara is the personification of all depravity and delusion, everything that makes us suffer in life.

The Buddha was taking a solo retreat in a cave. His attendant and student, the Venerable Ananda, would go out begging for alms, and upon returning would divide his offerings into two, one part for him and one for the Buddha. One morning as the Buddha was sitting inside the cave in meditation, the Venerable Ananda, sitting outside of the cave, saw someone approaching. Ananda had an inkling that this was someone very familiar. It was Mara!

Ananda wanted to hide somewhere, so that Mara, not seeing anyone, would not approach the cave and disturb the Buddha. But it was too late. Mara walked up to Ananda and asked, 'Venerable Ananda, is your teacher here?' Ananda wanted to lie and say, 'No, the Buddha is not here. The Buddha went to ...' some kind of meeting, conference, or something! But lying is not appropriate for a monk, so he finally said, 'Why do you ask?'

Mara said, 'I want to visit the Buddha.' Ananda responded rather scornfully, 'Go away! You're not a friend of the Buddha. You're his enemy. Don't you remember how you tried to discourage the Buddha from awakening under the Bodhi tree and the Buddha defeated you terribly? The Buddha won't see you.'

When Mara heard that, he laughed, 'Ha, ha, ha. Really? Your Buddha has enemies? I thought he said he doesn't have any enemies. Why is it that he has an enemy now?'

Ananda was dumbstuck. So he went into the cave to ask the Buddha if he wanted to see Mara. Ananda was hoping the Buddha would refuse. But when he heard who was waiting outside, the Buddha said, 'Mara? Let him in.' Ananda was really disappointed, but he was obliged to go out and let Mara in.

When Mara entered, the Buddha stood up and welcomed Mara as if he were an old friend. He invited Mara to sit down in a distinguished place and asked Ananda to bring tea and water for Mara to drink. Ananda was really unhappy about it. He would be happy to get tea for the Buddha two hundred times a day. But for Mara, Ananda didn't want to do it at all. But he went and got tea for Mara, hoping that Buddha and Mara would have a short conversation. In fact, the conversation ended up being very long.

Buddha and Mara spoke as if they were the best of friends. Buddha said, 'Mara, how has it been for you? How are you doing?' Mara said, 'Not very well.' 'What happened?' the Buddha asked.

Mara answered, 'My disciples aren't listening to me anymore. They used to do everything I told them to, but nowadays they want to rebel. All my generals, all my soldiers, all my disciples, they want to practice mindfulness. They want to practice walking meditation. They want to practice eating in silence. They want to protect the Earth. I don't know who got to them. Dear Buddha, I'm just so tired of being Mara; I want to be someone else. Don't think that being Mara is all wild parties, fun, and games.'

The Buddha laughed. 'You think being a Buddha is such a lark? Do you know that people say things that I have never said and then they say it is I who said that? They do things that I have never done or encouraged them to do, but they say that I encouraged them to do those things.

'I let go of my exalted reputation, my princely position, and an endless availability of sensual pleasures. I abandoned my throne, my beautiful wife and baby, future children, and wealth, all so that I could realize liberation. But now people come to the temple to pray and plead with me to give them all the very things I have renounced! They don't ask for peace or joy; they just ask for lots of money, power, or for their children to have good grades on their exams.

'They build a big house and they say it's my house. But it's only a place where people come to pass by and offer food, bananas, sweet rice, and money, so that they can have more money to spend on themselves. They make statues of me and they stick all their money on my body. When they celebrate my birthday, they put my statue up on top of a car and they drive mindlessly through the city while my body rocks from side to side. I didn't ever want to be riding on a car. So don't think that being Buddha is lucky. Do you want to exchange places?'

Ananda was terrified that Mara would agree, but luckily, he didn't. Then the Buddha said, 'Mara, you do your job. Do your job the best you can. I'll do my job. Nothing is easy all the time. I know being Mara is very difficult. But being a Buddha has its difficulties too. Each one of us has to play our part wholeheartedly.'

Every life has its trials and tribulations. We can navigate them more skillfully when we don't waste time and energy shooting ourselves with a second arrow—such as dwelling on how much greener the grass in our neighbor's yard looks, compared to ours.

5

FIVE PRACTICES
FOR NURTURING
HAPPINESS

~

We don't have to wait for the end of all suffering before we can be happy. Happiness is available to us right here and right now. But we may need to change our idea of happiness. Our idea of happiness may itself be the main obstacle keeping us from true happiness. There are oysters living in the depths of the sea, and they don't have any eyes; they have never seen the blue sky or the stars. We have eyes. We can see the beautiful sky above us, but we often don't appreciate what we have. Most of the time we just ignore it. There are more conditions of happiness available than you and I can count, many more than it takes to make us happy in the here and the now. If you're able to read a book, to read and understand these words, you are already much luckier than many people.

## The Difference Between Joy And Happiness

We can experience both joy and happiness, and Buddhist teachings do make a distinction between the two. In joy, there is still some element of excitement. Think of a person walking in the desert who has run out of drinking water. If suddenly that person sees that there is an oasis ahead—trees with beautiful shade and a lake of fresh water—he will feel joy. When he arrives at the lake and actually cups the water and drinks, this is happiness. You can experience both.

The method here is simple. Breathing in, bring your mind home to your body. Establish yourself in the here and the now and recognize what is around you. Then joy and happiness arise easily, from your recognition of all the positive elements available right now.

## Why The Buddha Kept Meditating

When I was a young monk, I wondered why the Buddha kept practicing mindfulness and meditation even after he had already become a Buddha. Now I find the answer is plain enough to see. Happiness is impermanent, like everything else. In order for happiness to be extended and renewed, you have to learn how to feed your happiness. Nothing can survive without food, including happiness; your happiness can die if you don't know how to nourish it. If you cut a flower but you don't put it in some water, the flower will wilt in a few hours. Even if happiness is already manifesting, we have to continue to nourish it. This is sometimes called conditioning, and it's very important. We can condition our bodies and minds to happiness with the five practices of letting go, inviting positive seeds, mindfulness, concentration, and insight.

## The First Practice! Letting Go

The first method of creating joy and happiness is to cast off, to leave behind. There is a kind of joy that comes from letting go. Many of us are bound to so many things. We believe these things are necessary for our survival, our security, and our happiness. But many of these things—or more precisely, our beliefs about their utter necessity—are really obstacles for our joy and happiness.

Sometimes you think that having a certain career, diploma, salary, house, or partner is crucial for your happiness. You think you can't go on without it. Even when you have achieved that situation, or are with that person, you continue to suffer. At the same time, you're still afraid that if you let go of that prize you've attained, it will be even worse; you will be even more miserable without the object you are clinging to. You can't live with it, and you can't live without it.

If you come to look deeply into your fearful attachment, you will realize that it is in fact the very obstacle to your joy and happiness. You have the capacity to let it go. Letting go takes a lot of courage sometimes. But once you let go, happiness comes very quickly. You won't have to go around searching for it.

Imagine you're a city dweller taking a weekend trip out to the countryside. If you live in a big metropolis, there's a lot of noise, dust, pollution, and odors, but also a lot of opportunities and excitement. One day, a friend coaxes you into getting away for a couple of days. At first you may say, 'I can't. I have too much work. I might miss an important call.' But finally he convinces you to leave, and an hour or two later, you find yourself in the countryside. You see open space. You see the sky, and you feel the breeze on your cheeks. Happiness is born from the fact that you could leave the city behind. If you hadn't left, how could you experience that kind of joy? You needed to let go.

## Releasing Your Cows

One day the Buddha was sitting with some of his monks in the woods. They had just come back from an almsround and were ready to share a mindful lunch together. A farmer passed by, looking distraught.

He asked the Buddha, 'Monks, have you seen some cows going by here?'

'What cows?' the Buddha responded.

'Well,' the man said. 'I have four cows and I don't know why, but this morning they all ran away. I also have two acres of sesame. This year the insects ate the entire crop. I have lost everything: my harvest and my cows. I feel like killing myself.' The Buddha said, 'Dear friend, we have been sitting here almost an hour and we have not seen any cows passing by. Maybe you should go and look in the other direction.' When the farmer was gone, the Buddha looked at his friends and smiled knowingly. 'Dear friends, you are very lucky,' he said. 'You don't have any cows to lose.'

I knew a rich woman living in New York City who purchased a piece of land adjacent to her building. She wanted to build a huge apartment complex on the land and then sell it so she could make a lot of money. A friend came to visit her and stood looking out the window. It had a beautiful view of the George Washington Bridge and a lot of blue sky. The friend turned to the woman who had bought the land and said, 'Don't build the apartment complex. If you do, you won't have this beautiful view anymore. Your neighbors won't have a view anymore. You'll no longer see the blue sky and the river. You only need to stand here and look and already you can have happiness. What is the use of having more money and losing all that beauty and happiness?' The woman was able to hear this and changed her plans for the building, releasing one big cow, thanks to the wise counsel of a friend.

One of the biggest cows that we have is our narrow idea of happiness. You may suffer just because of your idea; and you continue to suffer until, one day, you are capable of releasing the idea and right away you feel happy.

A whole country can be caught in a single cow. A nation of

hundreds of millions may believe that such-and-such ideology is crucial for the country to become a big power in the world, and that superpower status is essential to the people's happiness. So they invest everything in that ideology, and insist it is the best way, the only way. Countries can hold on to their cows for hundreds of years, and during that time the people suffer a lot. Then finally one day, the country may be open to change and discover that it actually works better and creates more happiness when it's run a different way. Every one of us has an idea of happiness that can become too entrenched, too rigid. Every one of us has cows to be released.

Consider practicing to release your cows. Take a piece of paper and write down the names of your cows, the things you think of as crucial for your well-being. Perhaps this week you can start by releasing just one, perhaps two. Or perhaps each one takes a year or more. The more cows you release, the more joyful and happy you become.

## The Story Of Badhiya

There is a story about a cousin of the Buddha whose name was Badhiya. He was governor of a province in the kingdom of Shakya, in present-day India. One day a number of his friends who were monks and students of the Buddha came to him and invited him to join their community. He hesitated. As a governor, he had at his command many soldiers, a lot of money, and a very powerful position. But finally his friends persuaded him. He left it all behind and came empty-handed into the forest, where he was ordained by the Buddha as a monk. He didn't have a fancy house to live in anymore. He only had three robes, one bowl, and a sitting mat.

One night Badhiya was meditating at the foot of a tree. Suddenly, he uttered the words, 'Oh my happiness, oh my happiness.' It happened that another monk was sitting nearby. The other monk thought that Badhiya regretted having abandoned his position as governor. So in the early morning that monk went to the Buddha and reported to him, 'Dear teacher, late last night I was sitting in meditation. Suddenly I heard the monk Badhiya exclaiming, "Oh my happiness, oh my happiness." I think he has some problem.'

The Buddha sent his attendant to invite Badhiya to come. In front of a group of monks the Buddha said, 'Badhiya, is it true that last night during sitting meditation you pronounced two times the sentence, "Oh my happiness, oh my happiness"?' Badhiya said, 'Yes, noble teacher, I did pronounce that sentence twice.'

'Could you explain to us why you have pronounced these three words during the night?' the Buddha asked.

Badhiya said, 'Dear teacher, when I was a governor my palace was guarded by hundreds of soldiers. But I was still very afraid. I was afraid robbers would come and kill me or at least take away all my valuables. So day and night I lived in fear. But last night I realized that now I have nothing to lose. I was sitting out in the forest at the foot of a tree, and never in my life have I felt so safe. Nobody wants to kill me anymore because I have no power, no wealth, and no jewels for anyone to take. I have nothing. Yet I finally have everything. I am touching such a great happiness and freedom. That is why I have pronounced the words, "Oh my happiness, oh my happiness." If I have disturbed someone, I am sorry.'

## The Second Practice: Inviting Positive Seeds

We each have many kinds of 'seeds' lying deep in our consciousness. Those we water are the ones that sprout, come up into our awareness, and manifest outwardly. So in our own consciousness there is hell, and there is also paradise. We are capable of being compassionate, understanding, and joyful. If we pay attention only to the negative things in us, especially the suffering of past hurts, we are wallowing in our sorrows and not getting any positive nourishment. We can practice appropriate attention, watering the wholesome qualities in us by touching the positive things that are always available inside and around us. That is good food for our mind.

One way of taking care of our suffering is to invite a seed of the opposite nature to come up. As nothing exists without its opposite, if you have a seed of arrogance, you have also a seed of compassion. Every one of us has a seed of compassion. If you practice mindfulness of compassion every day, the seed of compassion in you will become strong. You need only concentrate on it and it will come up as a powerful zone of energy. Naturally, when compassion comes up, arrogance goes down. You don't have to fight it or push it down. We can selectively water the good seeds and refrain from watering the negative seeds. This doesn't mean we ignore our suffering; it just means that we allow the positive seeds that are naturally there to get attention and nourishment.

## The Third Practice: Mindfulness-Based Joy

Mindfulness helps us not only to get in touch with the suffering, so that we can embrace and transform it, but also to touch the wonders of life, including our own body. Then breathing in becomes a delight, and breathing out can also be a delight. You truly come to enjoy your breathing.

A few years ago, I had a virus in my lungs that made them bleed. I was spitting up blood. With lungs like that, it was difficult to breathe, and it was difficult to be happy while breathing. After treatment, my lungs healed and my breathing became much better. Now when I breathe, all I need to do is to remember the time when my lungs were infected with this virus. Then every breath I take becomes really delicious, really good.

When we practice mindful breathing or mindful walking, we bring our mind home to our body and we are established in the here and the now. We feel so lucky; we have so many conditions of happiness that are already available. Joy and happiness come right away. So mindfulness is a source of joy. Mindfulness is a source of happiness.

Mindfulness is an energy you can generate all day long through your practice. You can wash your dishes in mindfulness. You can cook your dinner in mindfulness. You can mop the floor in mindfulness. And with mindfulness you can touch the many conditions of happiness and joy that are already available. You are a real artist. You know how to create joy and happiness any time you want. This is the joy and the happiness born from mindfulness.

## Enjoying Sitting

Sitting meditation is also an opportunity to heal and to create moments of joy. It's not a time when you force yourself to sit there, waiting for the bell announcing the end of the sitting. That would be a waste. These are very rare, very precious moments of life, moments you will never get back again. Many people in the world don't have the time to sit and do nothing like that. They consider it to be uneconomical or a luxury; they say, 'time is money.' But we know that sitting can be very healing, very profitable in its own way. So we have to learn how to enjoy every moment of our sitting—how to breathe, how to sit, so that every moment of our sitting can be nourishing and healing.

## Enjoying Our Steps

Many of us are in a perpetual hurry, and we don't enjoy the steps we make. Every time we stop and bring the mind back to our breath and our step, we can produce a feeling of joy and peace, and get in touch with the wonders of life. Our body is a wonder. Our body is like a flower; it's a wonder of life. There are so many wonders of life around us and inside us that we're unable to be in touch with because we're always in a hurry. We're looking for something, maybe for some happiness. So we miss the life all around us; we walk like zombies, staring down at our smartphones or lost in our thoughts. We don't enjoy our steps.

In Plum Village, we practice walking meditation with the Sangha, the community of practice. If someone were to ask, 'What's the purpose of walking meditation? What's the point? Why do you practice it?' There are several answers we can give. But for me the best answer is, 'Because I like it.' I enjoy every step; every step makes me happy. There's no use in doing walking meditation if you don't enjoy every step you make. It would be a waste of time.

It's the same with sitting meditation. If someone asks, 'What's the use of sitting and not doing anything?' The best answer is, 'Because I enjoy sitting.' If you can't produce peace and joy in sitting meditation, then it's of no use. It wouldn't help you even if you sat ten hours a day.

We have to learn *how* to sit so that we can produce peace and joy during the time of sitting. We have to learn how to walk so that we can enjoy every step. Walking on the planet Earth is a very wonderful thing to do. There are scientists who spend months out in space, far away from Earth. When they come back to Earth, they're so happy to take steps on our planet again.

This is about the quality of walking and sitting. We know that mindfulness and concentration can bring a higher quality to our steps, our breathing, and our sitting. Enlightenment is always enlightenment about something. You are *aware* that you are alive; that is already enlightenment. You are *aware* that you have a body; that is already enlightenment. You are *aware* that your feet are strong enough for you to enjoy walking; that is also enlightenment.

When you brush your teeth, you can choose to do it in mindfulness. You don't think of other things. You just focus your attention on brushing your teeth. You spend maybe two or three minutes brushing your teeth. You can produce the energy of joy and happiness during that time simply by being mindful of your teeth and of your brushing. When you go to the toilet, defecating or urinating, it's also possible to enjoy that time. Mindfulness can change everything by helping you to really be there and enjoy whatever you're doing.

Many of us have spent our lives pursuing material comforts

and affective comforts. We may find that we have succeeded—we have enough money and we have someone who loves and understands us; yet we're not happy. Perhaps it's because we aren't practicing the mindfulness that would help us recognize the many conditions of happiness that are there.

## Morning Verse For Happiness

When you wake up in the morning, the first thing to do is to breathe and to become aware that you have twenty-four brand-new hours to live. This is a gift of life.

After I was ordained as a novice monk, I had to memorize many short verses to help me practice mindfulness.

The first verse is:

*Waking up this morning I smile.*
*I have twenty-four hours to live.*
*I vow to live them deeply*
*and learn to look at the beings around me*
*with the eyes of compassion.*

There are four lines. The first line is for your in-breath. The second line is for your out-breath. The third line is for your in-breath again. The fourth line is for your out-breath. As you breathe, you use the verse to focus your attention on the meaning of the words. You want to live the twenty-four hours that are given you in such a way that peace, joy, and happiness are possible. You're determined not to waste your twenty-four hours, because you know those twenty-four hours are a gift of life, and you receive that gift every morning. That is mindfulness.

There are more than fifty such verses that a new monk or

nun has to memorize and practice throughout the day. When she brushes her teeth, she silently recites a verse. When he urinates, there is a verse to practice. When she puts on her robe, there is another verse for that. The practice of mindfulness means to be aware of everything you do in your daily life—to live more deeply every moment that is given you to live, so you won't waste your time and waste your life.

## Creating Happiness

We know how to nourish happiness with mindfulness. We get in touch with the wonderful elements of life in us and around us. We don't need to run around. We don't have to go looking into the future. The conditions are already there. With mindfulness we can discover the fact that the conditions of happiness we already have are sufficient, really much more than sufficient, and happiness is possible right now. When you walk, it can be a celebration. When you breathe with awareness, it's to celebrate. When we sit like that, we are celebrating; we're celebrating life.

Just as we may have many small sorrows that mindfulness can help us release, we also have a multitude of small moments of happiness that we can savor and extend. Whether you drink a cup of tea or take a walk or just sit down and look, you can create happiness during that time. People complain that they don't have any happiness in life. We need to find the many small joys that life has to offer and help them grow.

There are many talented people with diplomas, degrees, and long titles. There are people who can invent revolutionary new machines and computer applications. We may like to ask them, 'Can you create a moment of happiness?' If you know how to do this, you can create something truly beneficial.

To make a soup we need some water, some vegetables, some tofu, a little of this and a little of that. You can make a good soup with just a few simple ingredients; nothing fancy is needed. A small portion of happiness is a kind of soup. With a few ingredients, an open mind, and a little resourcefulness, we can make a moment of happiness for ourselves and for the person next to us. We can offer some of our tasty soup to someone else. If we know how to create a moment of happiness, we get to enjoy that happiness ourselves, and we can also double it by sharing it with another person. That is the art of happiness, tasting and delighting in the little happinesses of daily life.

I suggest you take a piece of a paper and write down all the conditions for happiness available to you right now. One page may not be enough. Two pages may not be enough. Three or four pages may not be enough. When we recognize all these elements, it's so easy to generate happiness.

### The Fourth Practice! Concentration

Concentration is born from mindfulness. Concentration has the power to break through, to burn away the afflictions that make you suffer and to allow joy and happiness to come in.

To stay in the present moment takes concentration. Worries and anxiety about the future are always there, ready to take us away. We can see them, acknowledge them, and use our concentration to return to the present moment.

When we have concentration, we have a lot of energy. We won't get carried away by visions of past suffering or fears about the future. We dwell stably in the present moment so we can get in touch with the wonders of life, and generate joy and happiness.

Concentration is always concentration on something. If you focus on your breathing in a relaxed way, you are already cultivating an inner strength. When you come back to feel your breath, concentrate on your breathing with all your heart and mind. Concentration is not hard labor. You don't have to strain yourself or make a huge effort. Happiness arises lightly and easily.

## The Fifth Practice: Insight

With mindfulness, we recognize the tension in our body, and we want very much to release it, but sometimes we can't. What we need is some insight.

Insight is seeing what is there. It is the clarity that can liberate us from afflictions such as jealousy or anger, and allow true happiness to come. Every one of us has insight, though we don't always make use of it to increase our happiness.

We may know, for example, that something (a craving, or a grudge) is an obstacle for our happiness, that it brings us anxiety and fear. We know this thing is not worth the sleep we're losing over it. But still we go on spending our time and energy obsessing about it. We're like a fish who has been caught once before and knows there's a hook inside the bait; if the fish makes use of that insight, he won't bite, because he knows he'll get caught by the hook.

Often, we just bite onto our craving or grudge, and let the hook take us. We get caught and attached to these situations that are not worthy of our concern. If mindfulness and concentration are there, then insight will be there and we can make use of it to swim away, free.

In springtime when there is a lot of pollen in the air, some of us have a hard time breathing due to allergies. Even when we aren't trying to run five miles and we just want to sit or lie down, we can't breathe very well. So in wintertime, when there's no pollen, instead of complaining about the cold, we can remember how in April or May we couldn't go out at all. Now our lungs are clear, we can take a brisk walk outside and we can breathe very well. We consciously call up our experience of the past to help ourselves treasure the good things we are having right now.

In the past we probably did suffer from one thing or another. It may even have felt like a kind of hell. If we remember that suffering, not letting ourselves get carried away by it, we can use it to remind ourselves, 'How lucky I am right now. I'm not in that situation. I can be happy'—that is insight; and in that moment, our joy, and our happiness can grow very quickly.

6

HAPPINESS
IS NOT AN
INDIVIDUAL MATTER

~

We've seen that our suffering is connected with the suffering of our ancestors, our loved ones, and with the planet itself, so we know our happiness is not an individual matter. If we are able to breathe happily, we can invite our ancestors to enjoy breathing in with our lungs. If we are able to enjoy walking, we can invite our ancestors to walk with our feet.

When a young person tells his parents, 'This is my body; this is my life. I can do what I want with it' he is only partly right. He doesn't see that he is the continuation of his parents and of his ancestors before that. This body is not yours alone. It is also the body of your ancestors. Your body is a collective product of your nation, of your people, of your culture, of your ancestors. So you are not strictly an individual. You are partly collective.

There are many people who have enormous suffering, overwhelming suffering, and they don't know how to end this suffering. For many people, this suffering starts at a very young age. So why don't schools teach us how to manage suffering? If your suffering is so great, you can't concentrate, you can't study, and you can't focus. The suffering of each of us affects others. The more we can teach each other about the art of suffering well, the less suffering there will be in the world overall and the more happiness.

## Borrowing Mindfulness

There are times when a case of suffering is so great, it needs recognition from more than just one person. We all need help sometimes when suffering threatens to overwhelm us. We can borrow the collective energy of mindfulness of a group of practitioners, in order to recognize and embrace the block of suffering in us. When suffering has become a seemingly impenetrable obstacle, we can learn how to draw on the support of others.

If we can take the time to sit together and allow the collective energy of mindfulness to recognize and embrace our pain, we become a drop of water flowing in the river of awakened energy and we feel much better. We may not have to do or even say anything. We just allow our pain to be embraced by the collective energy of mindfulness. Sometimes we may have to reach out more directly and ask for help. That can be very difficult. But other people do want to help, if we only ask them.

If we have loved ones who are suffering, one of the best things that we can do is to offer to sit or walk with them, and offer them our energy of mindfulness and peace. It can help calm them down and embrace their suffering, so that they can walk, sit, and breathe in mindfulness, and take care of the crying baby inside them.

## Being There For Another's Sorrows

When you love someone, you want to offer her something that can make her happy. According to this practice, the most precious thing that you can offer your beloved is your presence.

How can you love if you are not there? In order to love, you have to be there. To be there is a practice. It could be that very often your body is there but your mind is elsewhere. You're lost in your thinking, your sorrow, your fear; you're not really there for her. So breathe in and focus your attention on your in-breath. You are bringing your mind home to your body and you become present. Simply to be there is the most important part of the practice.

When you are truly there, you can go to the person you love, look into her eyes and say to her, 'I am here for you.' The most precious thing you can offer the person you love is your presence. It's not something you can buy in the supermarket.

## Collective Suffering, Collective Joy

When people come together and produce the energy of mindfulness, concentration, and compassion, it gives rise to a wholesome kind of collective consciousness. This is a good thing to consume. At one talk I gave in Germany, there were a thousand people listening peacefully, including four young mothers who were breast-feeding their babies. The infants were consuming the milk from their mothers and they were also consuming the collective energy of peace.

When the September 11, 2001, attacks happened, I was in California, about to give a public talk. Of course the whole American nation was shaken by the news. The energy of anger and fear was tremendous and I could feel it. It's very dangerous if we unconsciously allow that kind of energy to penetrate and to harm us.

So the talk I gave that night was about calming strong emotions. When a whole community is afraid or angry, their energy is very strong which can create a desire to strike back right away. But action pushed by the collective energy of anger and fear is not usually right action. We can start a devastating war very easily.

*No Mud, No Lotus*

## Taking Refuge In Oneself

When people around you are practicing compassion, they'll be wiser and happier, not only individually but also as a group. Combining our experiences and insights leads to a collective insight that can be wiser than the sum of its parts.

Without a community, it's harder for a person to change anything. If you work in a hospital or a clinic, or anyplace where you have to practice compassion with people in crisis on a daily basis, you know that having colleagues who support you in that practice creates a much more healing effect. A good environment allows the best things in us to manifest. A toxic environment can bring out the worst things in us.

Everyone needs a mindful community for support. We can join together to create a healing environment wherever we are. Our family, our classroom, and our workplace can all be mindful communities. When we come together and enjoy practicing mindful breathing together, we produce a collective energy of mindfulness and compassion that is wholesome and very strong. In our daily lives, many of us are in toxic environments of mutually reinforcing suspicion, competition, greed, and jealousy. We consume our environment as a kind of food, and its good or harmful elements seep into us.

You may find yourself in a negative environment you can't get out of due to the realities of family needs or financial constraints. In that case, you can be a force for positive change. Start by creating your own safe harbor, even if it's only one corner of a room or a desk. There are also wholesome communities online that you can join. Don't give up hope.

You can live in such a way that shows compassion is possible in any situation. Set an example, even if it's a small one; other people can learn from it. The best way to help others lessen their fear, craving, and violence is to show them there is another way. If love has degenerated into hate, it's possible for you to turn the garbage of that hate into a kind of compost to nourish the flower of love to bloom again.

## Collective Action

When a group comes together and commits to practicing mindfulness together—breathing together, walking together, doing some kind of good work together to lessen the suffering in the world—this is positive, collective action that can be very powerful. In the collective action, you can see the individual aspect. There are those who sit differently than others. There are some who focus more easily, some who need more support. In the collective we can see the individual, and in the individual there is the collective. There is no absolute individuality; there is no absolute collectivity.

Anything you can do to lessen suffering in your community and in the world is known in Buddhism as Right Action. When you go to the supermarket, you can make the choice whether to practice Right Action or not. There are items for sale that have been produced by children who have no chance to go to school. There are items that have been made with materials that can be harmful. We are part of the collective whole, and even these individual decisions about what to consume affect the collective consciousness.

I remember one day I went with some children to a hardware store. We visited all the items in the store. We only needed a few nails for a project, and we agreed with each other in advance that we wouldn't buy anything else. We spent over an hour in the store, learning about the origin and the effect of each item sold and not buying anything but a handful of nails. We did that as a special group activity. You don't have to spend an hour every time you want to buy one item; but you can feel much happier when you know the things in your home are not infused with the pain of child laborers or a poisoned field.

## The Whole World Is Our Territory

We may think we are only responsible for our own suffering and happiness, but our happiness increases the world's happiness and our suffering is the world's suffering. In Vietnam, there is a Buddhist folktale about Mara, the personification of distraction, attachment, and despair—the devilish character that Ananda tried to keep away from the Buddha's cave.

They say that before the Buddha's enlightenment, when the world was under the reign of Mara, there was a lot of war and violence. People suffered enormously. But they reminded themselves, 'If there's Mara, there is the Buddha. We don't need to worry. The Buddha will appear eventually.'

On the day the Buddha became enlightened, he sat very quietly. Mara said, 'Who is this guy sitting so quietly?' Mara didn't disturb the Buddha; he just allowed the Buddha to sit. After sitting in meditation, the Buddha stood up and walked mindfully, freely, and peacefully. Mara asked, 'Who are you? Why are you here?'

The Buddha said, 'I see that this Earth is a beautiful place; the scenery is lovely. The early morning is beautiful. The afternoon and the evening are beautiful. I see these wonders and it makes me so happy. I don't need to have any possessions or wealth. I don't need anything. All I need is the opportunity to sit still and to be able to walk on this beautiful planet.'

Mara thought that this wasn't a bad request. 'Okay, you can sit as much as you want, walk as much as you want,' he said.

A few days later, the Buddha asked, 'I have a few friends. Actually I have 1,250 friends, and they all want to sit; they all want to walk in mindfulness. Can we have an area here to sit and walk mindfully and peacefully?' Mara said, 'Sure, if you sit and walk, that's fine. How much space do you want to have for practicing sitting meditation and walking meditation?'

Back then they didn't have fancy measuring devices. The Buddha said, 'I have three robes. If you agree, I'll take off my outer robe and I'll throw it up in the sky as high as I can. The shadow cast on the Earth by my robe is the land I want to have for sitting, walking, and living mindfully.'

Mara said, 'Well, the most it could be is just a few miles. Okay.' The Buddha rolled up his robe and threw it up in the sky. The robe went high, high, high up. Then it opened, and the shadow of the robe covered the whole planet.

From then on, the Buddha and his students walked all over the Earth, practicing compassion and mindfulness and helping people suffer less. We all have the right to do the same on this planet, lessening suffering and increasing happiness. This Earth is not just the territory of Mara, but also the territory of the Buddha.

## The Art Of Happiness

The essence of our practice can be described as transforming suffering into happiness. It's not a complicated practice, but it requires us to cultivate mindfulness, concentration, and insight. It requires first of all that we come home to ourselves, that we make peace with our suffering, treating it tenderly, and looking deeply at the roots of our pain. It requires that we let go of useless, unnecessary sufferings, release the second arrow, and take a closer look at our idea of happiness. Finally, it requires that we nourish happiness daily, with acknowledgment, understanding, and compassion for ourselves and for those around us. We offer these practices to ourselves, to our loved ones, and to the larger community. This is the art of suffering and the art of happiness. With each breath, we ease suffering and generate joy. With each step, the flower of insight blooms.

PRACTICES
FOR
HAPPINESS

~

## One:
## The Sixteen Breathing Exercises

These exercises are taken from the Anapanasati Sutra on mindful breathing. There are sixteen exercises in all. The first four are to take care of our body. The second set of four exercises takes care of our feelings. The third set of four focuses on the mind, and the fourth set focuses on objects of the mind.

Although the first set of exercises is primarily for taking care of and healing the body, when you do them you also produce pleasure, freedom, and joy in your mind at the same time, because the body is always manifesting together with feelings and the mind.

The mind can be described as being made up of particles—like the drops of water in a river—called mental formations. Each drop of water in the river of the mind is a mental formation. Mindfulness, concentration, loving kindness, and insight are all mental formations.

The fourth set focuses on objects of mind because mental formations always have their objects. To be angry is always to be angry at something. To love means to love someone or something.

| BREATHING EXERCISE / SET 1 | DESCRIPTION |
|---|---|
| Breathing in, I am aware of my in-breath. Breathing out, I am aware of my out-breath. | This very simple exercise can help you to let go of your thinking, your worries, and your fear. It gives you a lot of freedom right away. |

| | |
|---|---|
| Breathing in, I follow my in-breath all the way through. Breathing out, I follow my out-breath all the way through. | Follow your in-breath and out-breath closely, being aware of each one all the way through as if following a line with your finger. Breathing like that, not only are you aware of your breath, you are fully concentrating on that breath. |
| Breathing in, I am aware of my whole body. Breathing out, I am aware of my whole body. | This exercise brings body and mind together. We are truly established in the here and now, living our life deeply in this moment. |
| Breathing in, I calm my body. Breathing out, I calm my body. | This exercise is to release the tension in the body. Releasing is a source of happiness. |

| BREATHING EXERCISE / SET 2 | DESCRIPTION |
|---|---|
| Breathing in, I feel joy. Breathing out, I feel joy. | We can make use of mindfulness to bring in a feeling of joy any place, any time. |
| Breathing in, I feel happy. Breathing out, I feel happy. | Mindfulness helps us to recognize the many conditions of happiness we already have. |
| Breathing in, I am aware of a painful feeling. Breathing out, I am aware of a painful feeling. | When a painful feeling or emotion manifests, we should be there to take care of it. With mindfulness, we recognize the pain, embrace it, and bring relief. |

| | |
|---|---|
| Breathing in, I calm my painful feeling. Breathing out, I calm my painful feeling. | This exercise calms body and mind, and makes them peaceful. Body, mind, feelings, and breath are unified. |

| BREATHING EXERCISE / SET 3 | DESCRIPTION |
|---|---|
| Breathing in, I am aware of my mind. Breathing out, I am aware of my mind. | The river of mind flows day and night. Mental formations take turns manifesting. We are there and recognize them as they arise, stay for some time, and go away. |
| Breathing in, I make my mind happy. Breathing out, I make my mind happy. | We gladden the mind by inviting the good seeds to manifest. The landscape of the mind becomes pleasant. |
| Breathing in, I concentrate my mind. Breathing out, I concentrate my mind. | We maintain awareness on the object of our concentration. Only concentration can liberate us from notions and bring insight. |
| Breathing in, I liberate my mind. Breathing out, I liberate my mind. | With this exercise, we untie all the knots in the mind. Calmly, we observe the mind in all its subtlety, to free ourselves from such obstacles as sadness and anxiety about the past and the future, and confusion and misperception in the present. |

| BREATHING EXERCISE / SET 4 | DESCRIPTION |
|---|---|
| Breathing in, I observe the impermanent nature of all dharmas. Breathing out, I observe the impermanent nature of all dharmas. | The concentration on impermanence is a deep and wonderful path of meditation. It's a fundamental recognition of the nature of all that exists. Everything is in endless transformation and all things are without an independent self. |
| Breathing in, I observe the disappearance of desire. Breathing out, I observe the disappearance of desire. | Seeing the true nature of our desire and the objects of desire, we know that happiness doesn't lie in attaining those objects or in our hopes for future accomplishments. We observe clearly the impermanent nature of all things, their coming into being and fading away. |
| Breathing in, I observe cessation. Breathing out, I observe cessation. | Cessation means cessation of all the erroneous notions and ideas that keep us from directly experiencing the ultimate reality, and cessation of the suffering that's born from ignorance. Then we can be in touch with the wonderful true nature of the way things are. |

| Breathing in, I observe letting go. Breathing out, I observe letting go. | This exercise helps us look deeply to give up desire and attachment, fear and anger. We don't let go of reality. We let go of our wrong perceptions about reality. The more we let go, the happier we become. |
| --- | --- |

## The First set of Four Exercises

The first exercise is mindfulness of our breathing. 'Breathing in, I know I'm breathing in. Breathing out, I know I'm breathing out.' Bringing our awareness to our breathing, we stop all the thinking and focus only on our in-breath and out-breath.

The second exercise is 'Breathing in, I follow my in-breath all the way through. Breathing out, I follow my out-breath all the way through. This exercise focuses and concentrates the mind. We follow our in-breath and out-breath from beginning to end without interruption.

The third exercise is 'Breathing in, I'm aware of my body. Breathing out, I'm aware of my body.' With this exercise we remember we have a body and we bring our awareness to our body, reuniting body and mind. As you breathe in and out, becoming aware of your body, you may notice tension and pain in your body. You have allowed tension and strain to accumulate in your body, and that may be the starting place for any number of illnesses. That's why you're motivated to release these tensions; and it's further applied in the fourth exercise of mindful breathing: 'Breathing in, I release the tension in my body. Breathing out, I release the tension in my body.' Or: 'Breathing in, I calm my body. Breathing out, I calm my body.' We may need some insight that can help us release the tension and calm the body.

The Second Set of Four Exercises

With the fifth exercise you go from the realm of the body to the realm of feeling and you generate joy. 'Breathing in, I'm aware of the feeling of joy.' A mindfulness practitioner is able to generate joy and happiness. It's not so hard. There's a little difference between joy and happiness. Joy still has some of the element of excitement or anticipation in it. In happiness, there is ease and freedom.

The French have a song they like to sing, 'Qu'est-ce qu'on attend pour etre heureux?' (What are you waiting for in order to be happy?) You can be happy right here and right now. When you bring your mind home to your body, you're established in the present moment, and you become aware of the many wonders of life that are there, in and around you. With so many conditions of happiness available, you can easily create a feeling of joy, a feeling of happiness. Each exercise makes the next one possible.

So the fifth and the sixth exercises represent the art of happiness-how to generate joy and happiness for the sake of your enjoyment and your healing. The next two exercises are to recognize and take care of the pain that is there.

The seventh is 'Breathing in, I'm aware of the painful feeling in me.' When a painful feeling arises, the practitioner knows how to use mindfulness to handle it. You don't allow the painful feeling to overwhelm you or push you to react in a way that creates suffering for yourself and for others.

'Breathing in, I'm aware of the painful feeling in me. Breathing out, I'm aware of the painful feeling in me.' This is an art. We have to learn it, because most of us don't like to be with our pain. We're afraid of being overwhelmed by the pain, so we always seek to run away from it. There's loneliness, fear, anger, and despair in us. Mostly we try to cover it up by consuming. There are those of us who go and look for something to eat. Others turn on the television. In fact, many people do both at the same time. And even if the TV program isn't interesting at all, we don't have the courage to turn it off, because if we turn it off, we have to go back to ourselves and encounter the pain inside. The marketplace provides us with many items to help us in our effort to avoid the suffering inside.

According to this teaching and practice, we do the opposite: we go home to ourselves and take care of the pain. The way to go home without fear of being overwhelmed by the pain is by practicing mindful walking or mindful breathing to generate the energy of mindfulness. Fortified with that energy, we recognize the painful feeling inside and embrace it tenderly. We lullaby the crying baby. Just as the third exercise is 'aware of the body' and the fourth is 'calming the body,' the seventh exercise is to be aware of the painful feeling and the eighth is to embrace, calm, and soothe the pain. All of the first eight exercises are simple, and are easy enough for us to practice in daily life.

The Third Set of Four Exercises

The ninth exercise is: 'Breathing in, I am aware of the activities of my mind. Breathing out, I'm aware of the activities of my mind.' We continue to breathe mindfully and we recognize mental formations when they arise. And we can call them by their true names, such as 'anger' or 'joy.'

The tenth is to 'gladden the mind—to get in touch with the wholesome seeds that are there in the soil of our mind and water them, so that they can manifest as mental formations or zones of energy that make us happy. We do this for our own benefit and for the benefit of our loved ones.

The eleventh exercise is 'concentrating our mind.' And the twelfth is 'liberating the mind.' Concentration, *samadhi* in Sanskrit, is a powerful force that you can generate to make a breakthrough, to see clearly what is there and understand its true nature. The object can be a pebble, a leaf, a cloud, or it can be your anger or fear. Anything can be the object of your concentration. I think scientists also practice concentration. In order to realize a deeper understanding of something, they have to concentrate totally on it. But the practice of concentration, as we are using it here, has the very specific aim and purpose of transforming the afflictions in us—the fear, the anger, the illusion—so that we can be free.

The Final Set of Four Exercises

The thirteenth exercise is the concentration on impermanence. With the insight of impermanence, we see the interdependent and selfless nature of all that exists—that nothing has a separate, independent self.

With the fourteenth exercise, we recognize the true nature of desire and see that everything is already in the process of coming into being and disintegrating. With this insight, we no longer hold on to any object of desire or see any phenomenon as a changeless separate entity.

With the fifteenth exercise, we look into the nature of our ideas and notions and release them. When we're no longer grasping at notions, we experience the freedom and joy that comes from the cessation of illusion.

The sixteenth exercise helps us further shed light on desire and attachment, fear and anxiety, hatred and anger, and let them go. Our tendency is to think that if we let go, we'll lose the things that make us happy. But the opposite is true. The more we let go, the happier we become. Letting go doesn't mean we let go of everything. We don't let go of reality. But we let go of our wrong ideas and wrong perceptions about reality.

## Two:
## The Six Mantras

The Six Mantras are ways to express love and compassion. They can be very effective in transforming suffering and producing happiness in a relationship with a loved one, a friend, or a colleague. Children can practice them too. You may start by first practicing the Six Mantras with yourself, because you can only love and understand another when you have practiced love and understanding for yourself.

A mantra is a magic formula. Every time you pronounce a mantra you can transform the situation right away; you don't have to wait. Learn it so you can recite it when the time is appropriate. What makes the mantra effective is your mindfulness and concentration. If you aren't mindful and concentrated when you recite the mantra, it won't work. We are all capable of being mindful and concentrated.

| MANTRA | DESCRIPTION |
|---|---|
| I am here for you. | This mantra is a practice, not a declaration. To love someone means to be there for that person. But first you have to be there for yourself. The practice is to produce your true presence. |
| I know you are there, and it makes me very happy. | This mantra is to acknowledge the presence of the person you love and to say that you are very happy that he or she is still alive and available to you. Everyone wants to be embraced by the mindful attention of the one they love. This mantra will make the other person happy right away. |
| I know you suffer, and that is why I am here for you. | This mantra is for you to practice when you see that the other person suffers. If you are a lover, you need to know what is happening to the person you love. If you are there for that person, you will notice when he or she suffers. |

| I suffer. Please help. | This mantra is for you to practice when you yourself suffer, and you believe the other person has caused your suffering. Go to that person with mindfulness and concentration and say the mantra. It may be a little bit difficult because you feel hurt. It takes a little training, but you can do it. |
|---|---|
| This is a happy moment. | The fifth mantra is for us to remember how lucky we are that we have so many conditions of happiness available in the here and the now. |
| You are partly right. | This mantra is to remind us that as human beings we have both positive and negative traits. Our head shouldn't be turned by praise, nor should we despair when we're criticized. |

### The First Mantra

The first mantra is 'I am here for you.' It's not difficult to practice. To love someone means to be there for him or for her. This is an art and a practice. If you don't have enough mindfulness and concentration, you can't be there one hundred percent for yourself or for the other person. With the practice of mindful breathing, mindful walking, mindful sitting, you can bring your mind home to your body and establish yourself fully in the here and now, restoring your true presence. When you love someone, you have to offer that person the best you have. The best thing we can offer another person is our true presence.

Before you can be there for someone else, you have to be there for yourself. So we practice this mantra first with ourselves. 'I am here for you' also means that I am here for myself. The mind goes home to the body and we become aware that we have a body. This is something we forget, especially when we're absorbed in our work.

The practice of breathing in and out and bringing your mind home to your body can be very pleasant. You enjoy your in-breath, your body, and your mind. This can already have an effect on the other person. That person may be lost in thinking or worries about the past or the future. When you are truly there and you produce the mantra powerfully, you help the other person to come back to himself or herself, to be present here and now.

The first definition of love is to be there. This is a practice. How can you love if you are not there? In order to love you have to be there, body and mind united. A true lover knows that the practice of mindfulness is the foundation of true love.

The Second Mantra

The second mantra is also very powerful and can create happiness for both of you at the same time. 'Darling, I know you are there, and I am very happy.' You have already produced your true presence, and so you are in a position to recognize the presence of another person, someone who is very precious to you. When you say, 'Darling, I know you are there,' you are also saying, 'Your presence is very precious to me and is crucial for my happiness.'

You can't make the second step unless you have made the first step. The first step is the first mantra. 'I am here. I recognize my presence. I offer my presence to you, my beloved one.' This is the best gift a lover can make to her beloved one. Nothing is more precious than your presence. You can buy things from the market. But no matter how expensive the things are that you buy for that person, nothing is as precious as your presence. With mindfulness you can make your presence fresher, more pleasant, more loving, and you can offer that wonderful presence to your beloved one and make happiness for both of you.

## The Third Mantra

The third mantra is needed when you notice that the other person suffers. The third mantra can help him suffer less right away. First you practice breathing, sitting, or walking to restore your presence. Then you are ready to go to him and say, 'Darling, I know you suffer, and that is why I am here for you.' This is true love. True love is made of mindfulness. Because you are mindful, you know that something isn't going well with the other person. If you're able to notice that, then you can do something to help: 'Darling, I know you suffer. That is why I am here for you.' Before you've even had a chance to do anything he will suffer less right away.

When you suffer and your beloved one ignores your suffering, then you suffer even more. But if the other person is aware of your suffering and offers his presence to you during these difficult moments, you suffer less right away. It doesn't take much time to bring some relief. This is a mantra that you can use in your relationships when the other person suffers.

## The Fourth Mantra

The fourth mantra is a little bit more difficult, especially when you have too much pride in you. The fourth mantra is for when you yourself suffer, and you believe that the other person has caused your suffering. This happens from time to time. If it had been another person who had said or done that to you, you would have suffered less. But it was the person you love the most who said or did that. That's why you suffer very deeply. You may have the impulse to punish her, because she has dared to make you suffer.

When we suffer we think that the other person has caused our suffering. 'She doesn't love me. So why do I have to love her?' Our natural tendency is to want to punish the other person. And the way we do that is to show her that 'I can survive very well without you.' This is an indirect way of saying: 'I don't need you.' But that's not true love. Many of us have made that mistake. I also have made that mistake.

But we learn. In fact, when we suffer we do need the other person. That's the commitment we made in the beginning of our relationship. You have to be true and faithful to that commitment. When you suffer, you should tell her that you suffer and that you need her help. But we tend to do the opposite. We want to show her that we don't need her. We prefer to lock ourselves in our room and cry instead of asking for help. There is pride in you. But in love, there is no place for pride. This is why we need the fourth mantra: 'Darling, I suffer; please help.'

It's so simple, yet it's so difficult. But if you can bring yourself to pronounce the mantra, you will suffer less right away. I guarantee it.

If the other person notices that something is wrong and asks, 'Darling, are you suffering?' and tries to comfort you, you may have the impulse to respond, 'Suffer? Why should I suffer?' But that's not true; you suffer deeply. If she tries to come close and put her hand on your shoulder, you may want to say, 'Leave me alone.' Many of us commit this kind of mistake.

The practice of the fourth mantra is the opposite. You have to recognize that you suffer. 'Darling, I suffer. I want you to know it. Please help.' In fact the formula is really a little bit longer: 'Darling, I suffer. I don't understand why you have said such a thing to me. I don't understand why you have done such a thing to me. I suffer. Please explain. I need your help.' This is true love. But if you say, 'I'm not suffering, I don't need your help,' that's not true love.

Please write the mantra on a piece of paper the size of a credit card and put it in your wallet. The next time you suffer and you believe that he or she is the cause of your suffering, remember to take it out and read it, and you will know exactly what to do.

According to this practice, you have the right to suffer twenty-four hours, but not more. That's the deadline. Then you have to practice the fourth mantra. If you can't go to the person, you can use your mobile phone, your computer, or you can write it down on a piece of paper and put it on her desk or somewhere she will see it. I'm sure that when you are able to bring yourself to write it down, you will suffer less right away.

The mantra can be split into three parts. The first part is, 'Darling, I suffer, and I want you to know.' That is sharing; you share your happiness and your suffering. 'Please explain to me why you did that to me, why you said that to me. I suffer.'

The second part is: 'I am doing my best.' It means I am a practitioner of mindfulness, so when I get angry I don't say or do anything that can cause damage to myself or to you. I am practicing mindful breathing, mindful walking, and looking deeply into my suffering, to find out the root of my suffering. I believe that you have caused my suffering. But because I'm a practitioner, I know I shouldn't be too sure of that. I'm looking to see whether my suffering has come from a wrong perception on my part. Maybe you didn't mean to say or do that. Since I'm a practitioner, I'm now doing my best to practice looking deeply to recognize my anger and embrace it tenderly.

'I am doing my best' is a kind of reminder, and it's also an invitation for the other person to do the same. When she gets the message, she might think: 'Oh, I didn't know he was suffering. What have I done, what have I said so that he suffers like that?' Then both of you will be practicing looking deeply, and if one of you discovers the cause, that person should communicate right away and apologize for his or her unskillfulness, so the other person doesn't have to continue to suffer. The second sentence invites both people to be aware of what is going on and to look deeply to see what is the real cause of the suffering.

The third sentence is: 'Please help.' This part can be a little bit difficult, but it's very important; it takes some courage. When we love each other, we need each other, especially when we suffer. Your suffering is her suffering. Her happiness is your happiness. Looking deeply into the situation, we may have an insight as to how we can reconcile and reestablish harmony between us.

The three sentences are: 'I suffer, and I want you to know it. I'm doing my best. Please help.' When you take the piece of paper from your wallet and read it, you will remember just what you need to do.

## The Fifth Mantra

The fifth mantra is 'This is a happy moment.' This isn't autosuggestion or wishful thinking. There are many conditions of happiness for us to enjoy if we are mindful enough to be aware of them. This mantra is to remind us both that we are very lucky to have so many conditions of happiness available in the here and the now. Sitting with him, walking with her, you may like to pronounce the fifth mantra, for us to remember how lucky we are to have so many conditions of happiness. If we don't enjoy them, we are not wise at all. Recognizing that this moment is a happy moment depends on your mindfulness. Only mindfulness can help you touch the many conditions of happiness that are available in the here and the now. There are more than enough conditions for both of you to be happy. So as you sit together, as you walk together, and have the opportunity to have some time together, breathe in mindfully and be aware of how lucky you are. It is mindfulness that makes the present moment into a wonderful moment, into a happy moment. The practitioner is an artist; she knows how to bring happiness into the here and the now, with her practice.

## The Sixth Mantra

The sixth mantra is perfect for dealing with the suffering that comes from the complexes: thinking we are equal to, worse than, or better than another person.

When someone congratulates you or criticizes you, you can use the sixth mantra: 'Darling, you are partly right.' This means that 'Your criticism or praise is only partly right, because I have both weaknesses and strengths in me. If you congratulate me, I shouldn't get lost and ignore the negative things in myself.'

When we see something beautiful in the other person, we tend to ignore the things that aren't so beautiful. As human beings we have both positive and negative qualities. So when your beloved one congratulates you, telling you that you are the very image of perfection, you can say, 'Darling, that is only partly true. You know that I have the other things in me too.' You retain your humility. You're not a victim of self-delusion, because you know that you're not perfect.

When the other person criticizes you or says you have nothing to offer or, that you're worthless, you can say the same thing, 'Darling, you are only partly right, because I do have good things in me too.'

## Three:
## Being Present With Strong Emotions

When a painful emotion comes up, stop whatever you're doing and take care of it. Pay attention to what is happening. The practice is simple. Lie down, put your hand on your belly, and begin to breathe. Or you may sit on a cushion or on a chair. Stop thinking, and bring your mind down to the level of the navel.

When you look at a tree in a storm, if you focus your attention on the top of the tree, you'll see the leaves and branches blowing wildly in the wind, and the tree will look so vulnerable, as though it could be broken at any time. But when you direct your attention down to the trunk of the tree, there's not so much movement. You see the stability of the tree, and you see that the tree is deeply rooted in the soil and can withstand the storm. When we experience a strong emotion, the mind is agitated like the top of the tree. We have to bring our mind down to the trunk, to the abdomen, and focus all our attention on the rise and fall of the abdomen.

Breathing in, you notice the rising of your abdomen. Breathing out, notice the falling of your abdomen. Breathe deeply and focus your attention only on your in-breath and out-breath. If there is anything to be aware of, it's that an emotion is only an emotion, and that you are much more than one emotion. You are body, feelings, perceptions, mental formations, and consciousness. The territory of your being is large. One emotion is very little. An emotion is something that comes and stays for a while and eventually goes away. If during the time of the emotion, you have that insight, that insight will save you.

You don't have to die just because of one emotion.

We shouldn't wait until the strong emotion comes to begin learning. That may be too late; the emotion may carry you away. But you can learn now. Then, if the day after tomorrow you have a strong emotion, you'll have confidence that you can handle the strong emotion.

## Four:
## Inviting The Bell

Inviting the bell to sound is inviting happiness to enter our bodies and take root there. Every time we hear the sound of the bell, we have the chance to practice mindful breathing, calm our body, and notice our happiness. We can invite all the cells in our body to join us in listening to the bell and allowing the sound of the bell to penetrate into us. Listening deeply, we know that our ancestors are fully present in every cell of our body. We listen in such a way that all our ancestors are listening at the same time. If we can be peaceful and joyful while listening, then all our ancestors will also experience peace and joy at the same time. It is possible to invite all our ancestors to join us in listening to the bell.

# Five:
# Metta

*Metta* meditation is a practice of cultivating understanding, love, and compassion by looking deeply, first for ourselves and then for others. Once we love and take care of ourselves, we can be much more helpful to others. Metta meditation can be practiced in part or in full. Just saying one line of the Metta meditation will already bring more compassion and healing into the world.

To love is, first of all, to accept ourselves as we actually are. That is why in this love meditation, ' Know thyself' is the first practice of love. When we practice this, we see the conditions that have caused us to be the way we are. This makes it easy for us to accept ourselves, including our suffering and our happiness at the same time.

Metta means loving kindness in Pali. We begin this with an aspiration:'May I be ...' Then we transcend the level of aspiration and look deeply at all the positive and negative characteristics of the object of our meditation, in this case, ourselves. The willingness to love is not yet love. We look deeply, with all our being, in order to understand. We don't just repeat the words, or imitate others, or strive after some ideal. The practice of love meditation is not autosuggestion. We don't just say, 'I love myself. I love all beings.' We look deeply at our body, our feelings, our perceptions, our mental formations, and our consciousness, and in just a few weeks, our aspiration to love will become a deep intention. Love will enter our thoughts, our words, and our actions, and we will notice that we have become 'peaceful, happy, and light in body and spirit; safe and free from injury; and free from anger, afflictions, fear, and anxiety.'

When we practice, we observe how much peace, happiness, and lightness we already have. We notice whether we are anxious about accidents or misfortunes, and how much anger, irritation, fear, anxiety, or worry are already in us. As we become aware of the feelings in us, our self-understanding will deepen. We will see how our fears and lack of peace contribute to our unhappiness, and we will see the value of loving ourselves and cultivating a heart of compassion.

In this love meditation, 'anger, afflictions, fear, and anxiety' refer to all the unwholesome, negative states of mind that dwell in us and rob us of our peace and happiness. Anger, fear, anxiety, craving, greed, and ignorance are the great afflictions of our time. By practicing mindful living, we are able to deal with them, and our love is translated into effective action.

This is a love meditation adapted from the Visuddhimagga (The Path of Purification) by Buddhaghosa, a fifth-century CE systematization of the Buddha's teachings.

To practice this love meditation, sit still, calm your body and your breathing, and recite it to yourself. The sitting position is wonderful for practicing this. Sitting still, you are not too preoccupied with other matters, so you can look deeply at yourself as you are, cultivate your love for yourself, and determine the best ways to express this love in the world.

*May I be peaceful, happy, and light in body and spirit.*
*May she be peaceful, happy, and light in body and spirit.*
*May he be peaceful, happy, and light in body and spirit.*
*May they be peaceful, happy, and light in body and spirit.*

*May I be safe and free from injury.*
*May she be safe and free from injury.*

*May he be safe and free from injury.*
*May they be safe and free from injury.*

*May I be free from anger, afflictions, fear, and anxiety.*
*May she be free from anger, afflictions, fear, and anxiety.*
*May he be free from anger, afflictions, fear, and anxiety.*
*May they be free from anger, afflictions, fear, and anxiety.*

Begin practicing this love meditation on yourself ('I'). Until you are able to love and take care of yourself, you cannot be of much help to others. After that, practice on others ('he/she,' 'they')—first on someone you like, then on someone neutral to you, then on someone you love, and finally on someone the mere thought of whom makes you suffer.

According to the Buddha, a human being is made of five elements, called *skandhas* in Sanskrit. They are: form (body), feelings, perceptions, mental formations, and consciousness. In a way, you are the surveyor, and these elements are your territory. To know the real situation within yourself, you have to know your own territory, including the elements within you that are at war with each other. In order to bring about harmony, reconciliation, and healing within, you have to understand yourself. Looking and listening deeply, surveying your territory, is the beginning of love meditation.

Begin this practice by looking deeply into your body. Ask: How is my body in this moment? How was it in the past? How will it be in the future? Later, when you meditate on someone you like, someone neutral to you, someone you love, and someone you hate, you also begin by looking at his physical aspects. Breathing in and out, visualize his face; his way of walking, sitting, and talking; his heart, lungs, kidneys, and all the organs in his body, taking as much time as you need to bring these details into awareness. But always start with yourself. When you see your own five skandhas clearly, understanding and love arise naturally, and you know what to do and what not to do to take care of yourself.

Look into your body to see whether it is at peace or is suffering from illness. Look at the condition of your lungs, your heart, your intestines, your kidneys, and your liver to see what the real needs of your body are. When you do, you will eat, drink, and act in ways that demonstrate your love and your compassion for your body. Usually you follow ingrained habits. But when you look deeply, you see that many of these habits harm your body and mind, so you work to transform your habits in ways conducive to good health and vitality.

Next, observe your feelings—whether they are pleasant, unpleasant, or neutral. Feelings flow in us like a river, and each feeling is a drop of water in that river. Look into the river of your feelings and see how each feeling came to be. See what has been preventing you from being happy, and do your best to transform those things. Practice touching the wondrous, refreshing, and healing elements that are already in you and in the world. Doing so, you become stronger and better able to love yourself and others.

Then meditate on your perceptions. The Buddha observed, 'The person who suffers most in this world is the person who has many wrong perceptions, and most of our perceptions are erroneous.' You see a snake in the dark and you panic, but when your friend shines a light on it, you see that it is only a rope. You have to know which wrong perceptions cause you to suffer. Please write beautifully the sentence, 'Are you sure?' on a piece of paper and tape it to your wall. Love meditation helps you learn to look with clarity and serenity in order to improve the way you perceive.

Next, observe your mental formations, the ideas and tendencies within you that lead you to speak and act as you do. Practice looking deeply to discover the true nature of your mental formations—how you are influenced by your individual consciousness and also by the collective consciousness of your family, ancestors, and society. Unwholesome mental formations cause so much disturbance; wholesome mental formations bring about love, happiness, and liberation.

Finally, look at your consciousness. According to Buddhism, consciousness is like a field with every possible kind of seed in it: seeds of love, compassion, joy, and equanimity; seeds of anger, fear, and anxiety; and seeds of mindfulness. Consciousness is the storehouse that contains all these seeds, all the possibilities of whatever might arise in your mind. When your mind is not at peace, it may be because of the desires and feelings in your store consciousness. To live in peace, you have to be aware of your tendencies—your habit energies—so you can exercise some self-control. This is the practice of preventive health care. Look deeply into the nature of your feelings to find their roots, to see which feelings need to be transformed, and nourish those feelings that bring about peace, joy, and well-being.

You can continue with the following aspirations, first for yourself, then for others.

*May I learn to look at myself with the eyes of understanding and love.*

*May I learn to look at her with the eyes of understanding and love.*

*May I learn to look at him with the eyes of understanding and love.*

*May I learn to look at them with the eyes of understanding and love.*

*May I be able to recognize and touch the seeds of joy and happiness in myself.*

*May I be able to recognize and touch the seeds of joy and, happiness in her.*

*May I be able to recognize and touch the seeds of joy and happiness in him.*

*May I be able to recognize and touch the seeds of joy and happiness in them.*

*May I learn to identify and see the sources of anger, craving, and delusion in myself.*

*May I learn to identify and see the sources of anger, craving, and delusion in her.*

*May I learn to identify and see the sources of anger, craving, and delusion in him.*

*May I learn to identify and see the sources of anger, craving, and delusion in them.*

'May I learn to look at myself with the eyes of understanding and love.' One time when we practiced love meditation in Plum Village a young laywoman said to me, 'When I meditated on my boyfriend, I found that I began to love him less. And when

I meditated on the person I dislike the most, I suddenly hated myself.' Before the meditation, her love for her boyfriend was so passionate that she was not able to see his shortcomings. During her practice, she began to see him more clearly and she realized that he is less perfect than she imagined. She began to love him in a way that had more understanding in it, and therefore it was deeper and healthier.

She also had fresh insights into the person she disliked the most. She saw some of the reasons he was like that, and she saw how she had caused him to suffer by reacting to him harshly.

Again, we begin with ourselves to understand our own true nature. As long as we reject ourselves and continue to harm our own body and mind, there's no point in talking about loving and accepting others. With mindfulness we will be able to recognize our habitual ways of thinking and the contents of our thoughts. We shine the light of mindfulness on the neural pathways in our mind so we can see them clearly.

Whenever we see or hear something, our attention can be appropriate or inappropriate. With mindfulness we can recognize which it is and release inappropriate attention and nurture appropriate attention. Appropriate mental attention, *yoniso manaskara* in Sanskrit, brings us happiness, peace, clarity, and love. Inappropriate attention, *ayoniso manaskara,* fills our mind with sorrow, anger, and prejudice. Mindfulness helps us practice appropriate attention and water the seeds of peace, joy, and liberation in us.

Next, we use mindfulness to illuminate our speech, so we can use loving speech and stop before we say anything that creates conflict for ourselves and others. Then we look into our physical actions. Mindfulness illuminates how we stand, sit, walk, smile, and frown, and how we look at others. We recognize which actions are beneficial and which bring harm.

Understanding of oneself and others is the key that opens the door of love and acceptance of oneself and others.

'May I be able to recognize and touch the seeds of joy and happiness in myself.' The soil of our mind contains many seeds, positive and negative. We are the gardeners who identify, water, and cultivate the best seeds. Touching the seeds of joy, peace, freedom, solidity, and love in ourselves and in each other is an important practice that helps us grow in the direction of health and happiness.

'May I learn to identify and see the sources of anger, craving, and delusion in myself.' We look deeply to see how these came about, what are their roots, and how long they have been there. We practice mindfulness in our daily lives to be aware that such poisons as craving, anger, delusion, arrogance, and suspicion are present in us. We can look and see how much suffering they have caused ourselves and others.

We need to master our own anger before we can help others to do the same. Arguing with others only waters the seeds of anger in us. When anger arises, return to yourself and use the energy of mindfulness to embrace, soothe, and illuminate it. Don't think you'll feel better if you lash out and make the other person suffer. The other person might respond even more harshly and anger will escalate. The Buddha taught that when anger arises, close your eyes and ears, return to yourself, and tend to the source of anger within. Transforming your anger is not just for your personal liberation. Everyone around you and even those more distant will benefit.

Look deeply at your anger, as you would look at your

own child. Don't reject it or hate it. The point of meditation is not to turn yourself into a battlefield, one side opposing the other. Conscious breathing soothes and calms the anger, and mindfulness penetrates it. Anger is just an energy, and all energies can be transformed. Meditation is the art of using one kind of energy to transform another.

*May I know how to nourish the seeds of joy in myself every day.*
*May I know how to nourish the seeds of joy in her every day.*
*May I know how to nourish the seeds of joy in him every day*
*May I know how to nourish the seeds of joy in them every day.*

*May I be able to live fresh, solid, and free.*
*May she be able to live fresh, solid, and free.*
*May he be able to live fresh, solid, and free.*
*May they be able to live fresh, solid, and free.*

*May I be free from attachment and aversion, but not be indifferent.*
*May she be free from attachment and aversion, but not be indifferent.*
*May he be free from attachment and aversion, but not be indifferent.*
*May they be free from attachment and aversion, but not be indifferent.*

These aspirations help us to water the seeds of joy and happiness that lie deep in our store consciousness. The notions we entertain about what will bring us happiness are just a trap. We forget that they are only ideas. Our idea of happiness can prevent us from being happy. When we believe that happiness should take a particular form, we fail to see the opportunities for joy that are right in front of us.

Happiness is not an individual matter; it has the nature of inter-being. When you are able to make one friend smile, her happiness will nourish you also. When you find ways to foster peace, joy, and happiness, you do it for everyone. Begin by nourishing yourself with joyful feelings. Practice walking meditation outside, enjoying the fresh air, the trees, and the stars in the night sky. What do you do to nourish yourself? It's important to discuss this subject with dear friends to find concrete ways to nourish joy and happiness. When you succeed in doing this, your suffering, sorrow, and painful mental formations will begin to transform.

'May I be able to live fresh, solid, and free.' 'Fresh' is a translation of the Vietnamese word for 'cool, without fever.' Jealousy, anger, and craving are a kind of fever. 'Solid' refers to stability. If you aren't solid, you won't be able to accomplish much. Each day you only need to take a few solid steps in the direction of your goal. Each morning, you rededicate yourself to your path in order not to go astray. Before going to sleep at night, take a few minutes to review the day. 'Did I live in the direction of my ideals today?' If you see that you took two or three steps in that direction, that is good enough. If you didn't, say to yourself, 'I'll do better tomorrow.' Don't compare yourself with others. Just look to yourself to see whether you are going in the direction you cherish. Take refuge in things that are solid. If you lean on something that isn't solid, you will fall down. A few Sanghas may not yet be solid, but usually taking refuge in a Sangha is a wise thing to do. There are Sangha members everywhere who are practicing earnestly.

'Freedom' means transcending the trap of harmful desires

and being without attachments—whether to an institution, a diploma, or a certain rank. From time to time we encounter people who are free and can do whatever is needed.

'Indifference.' When we are indifferent, nothing is enjoyable, interesting, or worth striving for. We don't experience love or understanding, and our life has no joy or meaning. We don't even notice the beauties of nature or the laughter of children. We are unable to touch the suffering or the happiness of others. If you find yourself in a state of indifference, ask your friends for help. Even with all its suffering, life is filled with many wonders.

'Free from attachment and aversion.' The kind of love the Buddha wanted us to cultivate is not possessive or attached. All of us, young and old, have a tendency to become attached. As soon as we are born, attachment to self is already there. In wholesome love relationships, there is a certain amount of possessiveness and attachment, but if it's excessive, both lover and beloved will suffer. If a father thinks he 'owns' his son, or if a young man tries to put restrictions on his girlfriend, then love becomes a prison. This is also true in relationships between friends, teachers, students, and so on. Attachment obstructs the flow of life. And without mindfulness, attachment always becomes aversion. Both attachment and aversion lead to suffering. Look deeply to discover the nature of your love, and identify the degree of attachment, despotism, and possessiveness in your love. Then you can begin untangling the knots. The seeds of true love—loving kindness, compassion, joy, and equanimity—are already there in our store consciousness. Through the practice of deep looking, the seeds of suffering and attachment will shrink and the positive seeds will grow. We can transform attachment and aversion and arrive at a love that is spacious and all-encompassing.

# Six:
# Deep Relaxation

When we fall down, we have physical pain. When we're sad, we call it emotional pain. But mind and body are not separate, and suffering is not just an emotion. We hold suffering in our body. The practice of deep relaxation is a way to acknowledge and soothe the suffering in the body and the suffering in the mind.

Deep relaxation begins with observing our bodies. You can start with your eyes. 'Breathing in, I'm aware of my eyes. Breathing out, I smile to my eyes with gratitude and love.' Then bring your awareness down to your nose, your mouth, your throat, and continue down to your toes. You're doing a scan of your body, not with an x-ray, but with a ray of mindfulness. You go through your whole body, bringing your awareness to each part. 'Breathing in, I'm aware of my heart. Breathing out, I smile to my heart with love.' My heart is essential to my well-being. It works nonstop and nourishes all the cells in my body. I'm so grateful to my heart. I get to rest and sleep, but my heart never stops. Yet I've done things to hurt my heart. I've drunk too much alcohol; I've smoked. I haven't been very kind to my heart.' As you breathe in and out and embrace your heart with mindfulness, you can see things like this. This kind of insight can transform and heal. You know exactly what you should consume and what you should not consume to be kind to your heart, which is an essential condition of your happiness. You go through all your organs, all the parts of your body in this way. This is the contemplation of the body in the body.

There's a basic text in Buddhism that teaches us how to meditate on our body. It's called the Kayagatasati Sutta,

Mindfulness of the Body in the Body. The body is an important object of meditation. It contains the cosmos, the Kingdom of God, the Pure Land of the Buddha, and our ancestors both spiritual and genetic. Meditating on the body we can get in touch with all these things and nourish our happiness and well-being as well as the happiness and well-being of those around us.

## Seven:
## The Five Mindfulness Trainings

The Five Mindfulness Trainings are guidelines for how to live our daily lives in a way that nourishes happiness and transforms ill-being. The Five Mindfulness Trainings are also the kind of thinking and acting that have the power to heal. You can recite them daily or monthly, alone or with a group, to renew your intentions and as inspiration to practice.

### The First Mindfulness Training: Reverence for Life

Aware of the suffering caused by the destruction of life, I am committed to cultivating the insight of interbeing, compassion, and learning ways to protect the lives of people, animals, plants, and minerals. I am determined not to kill, not to let others kill, and not to support any act of killing in the world, in my thinking, or in my way of life. Seeing that harmful actions arise from anger, fear, greed, and intolerance, which in turn come from dualistic and discriminative thinking, I will cultivate openness, nondiscrimination, and nonattachment to views in order to transform violence, fanaticism, and dogmatism in myself and in the world.

### The Second Mindfulness Training: True Happiness

Aware of the suffering caused by exploitation, social injustice, stealing, and oppression, I am committed to practicing generosity in my thinking, speaking, and acting. I am determined not to steal and not to possess anything that should belong to others;

and I will share my time, energy, and material resources with those who are in need. I will practice looking deeply to see that the happiness and suffering of others are not separate from my own happiness and suffering; that true happiness is not possible without understanding and compassion; and that running after wealth, fame, power, and sensual pleasures can bring much suffering and despair. I am aware that happiness depends on my mental attitude and not on external conditions, and that I can live happily in the present moment simply by remembering that I already have more than enough conditions to be happy. I am committed to practicing Right Livelihood so that I can help reduce the suffering of living beings on Earth and reverse the process of global warming.

The Third Mindfulness Training: True Love

Aware of the suffering caused by sexual misconduct, I am committed to cultivating responsibility and learning ways to protect the safety and integrity of individuals, couples, families, and society. Knowing that sexual desire is not love, and that sexual activity motivated by craving always harms myself as well as others, I am determined not to engage in sexual relations without true love and a deep, long-term commitment made known to my family and friends. I will do everything in my power to protect children from sexual abuse and to prevent couples and families from being broken by sexual misconduct. Seeing that body and mind are one, I am committed to learning appropriate ways to take care of my sexual energy and cultivating loving kindness, compassion, joy, and inclusiveness—which are the four basic elements of true love—for my greater happiness and the greater happiness of others. Practicing true love, we know that we will continue beautifully into the future.

The Fourth Mindfulness Training: Loving Speech and Deep Listening

Aware of the suffering caused by unmindful speech and the inability to listen to others, I am committed to cultivating loving speech and compassionate listening in order to relieve suffering and to promote reconciliation and peace in myself and among other people, ethnic and religious groups, and nations. Knowing that words can create happiness or suffering, I am committed to speaking truthfully, using words that inspire confidence, joy, and hope. When anger is manifesting in me, I am determined not to speak. I will practice mindful breathing and walking in order to recognize and to look deeply into my anger. I know that the roots of anger can be found in my wrong perceptions and lack of understanding of the suffering in myself and in the other person. I will speak and listen in a way that can help myself and the other person to transform suffering and see the way out of difficult situations. I am determined not to spread news that I do not know to be certain and not to utter words that can cause division or discord. I will practice Right Diligence to nourish my capacity for understanding, love, joy, and inclusiveness, and gradually transform anger, violence, and fear that lie deep in my consciousness.

The Fifth Mindfulness Training: Nourishment and Healing

Aware of the suffering caused by unmindful consumption, I am committed to cultivating good health, both physical and mental, for myself, my family, and my society by practicing mindful eating, drinking, and consuming. I will practice looking deeply into how I consume the Four Kinds of Nutriments, namely edible foods, sense impressions, volition, and consciousness. I am determined not to gamble, or to use alcohol, drugs, or any other products that contain toxins, such as certain websites, electronic games, TV programs, films, magazines, books, and conversations. I will practice coming back to the present moment to be in touch with the refreshing, healing, and nourishing elements in me and around me, not letting regrets and sorrow drag me back into the past nor letting anxieties, fear, or craving pull me out of the present moment. I am determined not to try to cover up loneliness, anxiety, or other suffering by losing myself in consumption. I will contemplate interbeing and consume in a way that preserves peace, joy, and well-being in my body and consciousness, and in the collective body and consciousness of my family, my society, and the Earth.

# Eight:
## Walking Meditation

In our daily lives we have the habit of running. We seek peace, success, and love—we are always on the run—and our steps are one means by which we run away from the present moment. But life is available only in the present moment; peace is available only in the present moment. Taking a step and taking refuge in your step, means to stop running. For those of us who are used to always running, it is a revolution to make a step and stop running. We make a step, and if we know how to make it, peace becomes available in that moment of touching the Earth with our feet. It would be a pity to let a whole day pass without enjoying walking on the Earth.

Usually, our in-breath tends to be a little shorter than our out-breath. When you breathe in, you may take two steps and say: 'I have arrived, I have arrived.' When you breathe out, you might like to take three steps and say: 'I am home, I am home, I am home.' 'Home' means being at home in the present moment where you can touch all the wonders of life. We should be able to walk with a lot of tenderness and happiness on this beautiful planet. 'I have arrived, I am home,' is not a statement, but a practice. Allow yourself to sink deeply into the here and the now, because life is possible only in the present, life is available only in the present moment, and you know that you have the capacity to touch life in the present moment, in the here and the now.

We may have lost our freedom and our sovereignty. We may allow ourselves to be pushed and pulled away from the here and the now. Now we have to resist the habit energy that pushes us to run. We have to recover our sovereignty and reclaim our freedom and walk like a free person on Earth. Freedom doesn't mean political freedom. It means freedom from the past, from the future, from our worries and our fear. Each step can help free us. We resist, we don't allow ourselves to be carried away anymore. We want to be free, because we know that without freedom, no happiness, no peace, will be possible. The Buddha said that freedom and solidity are the two characteristics of nirvana. Imagine someone who has no solidity and no freedom. That person can never be happy. Walking like this helps us to cultivate freedom and solidity, which will bring us well-being and happiness.

Let your steps follow your breath, not the other way around. Let your breathing be natural, never forced. Breathing in, if your lungs want two steps, then we can take exactly two steps. If you feel better with three steps then give yourself three steps while breathing in. When you breathe out, listen to your lungs. Whenever you feel that you want to take an extra step while breathing out, then allow yourself to have one more step breathing out. Every step should be enjoyable.

Sometimes it's helpful to practice in a park or some other beautiful, quiet place. This nourishes our spirit and strengthens our mindfulness. We walk slowly but not too slowly, so we don't stand out and make people feel uncomfortable. This is a kind of invisible practice. We can enjoy nature and our own serenity. When we see something we want to touch with our mindfulness—the blue sky, the hills, a tree, or a bird—we just stop, but while we do so, we continue breathing in and out mindfully.

Practice stopping while you're walking. If you can stop

while walking, then you'll be able to stop when doing your other daily activities, whether that is cleaning the kitchen, watering the garden, or eating breakfast.

If you suffer from depression, your depression won't be able to go away until you know how to stop. You've lived in such a way that depression has become possible. You've been running and not allowed yourself the time to rest, to relax, and to live your daily life deeply. Spending time each day doing mindful walking can help. Arrange your life so that you can do mindful walking every day. It's good to walk alone, but it's also good to practice walking meditation with the Sangha, to get support. You can ask a friend to go with you, or you can even take the hand of a child and walk with him or her.

We should be able to practice mindful breathing and walking everywhere—in our home, at work, at school, in a hospital, even in Congress. Some years ago we offered a retreat for Congresspeople in Washington D.C. And now there are a number of Congressmen who know how to practice walking meditation on Capitol Hill.

When you walk to the bus stop or from one room to another, make it into a walking meditation. Even if your surroundings are full of noise and agitation, you can still walk in rhythm with your breathing. Even in the commotion of a big city, you can walk with peace, happiness, and an inner smile. This is what it means to live fully in every moment of every day of your life. This is something that is possible to do.

Walking in walking meditation is walking just to enjoy walking. You don't have any desire to arrive anywhere. Walking and not arriving, that is the technique. And you enjoy every step you make. Every step brings you home to the here and the now. Your true home is the here and the now, because only in this moment, in this place, called the here and the now, is life possible. Every step you take should bring you back to peace, to the present moment.

According to Master Linji the miracle is not to walk on water or in thin air, but to walk on Earth. Walk in such a way that you become fully alive and joy and happiness are possible. That is the miracle that everyone can perform. I perform that miracle every time I walk; and you can too. If you have mindfulness, concentration, and insight then every step you make on this Earth is performing a miracle.

Dharmacharya Shantum Seth, a teacher ordained by Thich Nhat Hanh, offers teachings and shares the practice of Mindfulness meditation in different parts of India and the world. He also leads pilgrimages, 'In the Footsteps of the Buddha'.

Please visit: www.buddhapath.com or contact info@buddhapath.com

Ahimsa Trust represents Thich Nhat Hanh and his community in India. It is a volunteer driven, non-profit trust, working to create peace, in one's self and in the world. Ahimsa Trust organizes Days of Mindfulness and retreats/workshops across India, especially for educators.

Please visit www.ahimsatrust.org or contact ahimsa.trust@gmail.com

For worldwide contacts and teachings of Thich Nhat Hanh and his community, please visit www.plumvillage.org

Made in the USA
Columbia, SC
11 May 2018